COUSINS AND STRANGERS

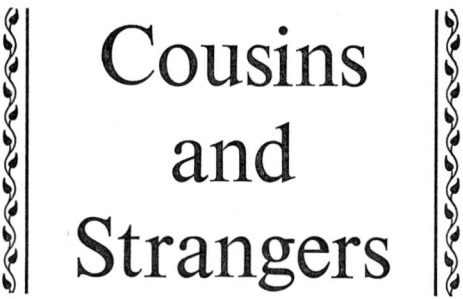

Cousins and Strangers

COMMENTS ON AMERICA BY

COMMONWEALTH FUND FELLOWS FROM BRITAIN

1946–1952

Edited by S. Gorley Putt

PUBLISHED FOR THE COMMONWEALTH FUND

BY HARVARD UNIVERSITY PRESS

Cambridge, Massachusetts

1956

Published for The Commonwealth Fund
By Harvard University Press

Distributed in Great Britain
By Geoffrey Cumberlege
Oxford University Press
London

MANUFACTURED IN THE UNITED STATES OF AMERICA

LIBRARY OF CONGRESS CATALOG CARD NO. 56–7901

Preface

WHEN THE IDEA of this anthology first took shape, it seemed like the promise of editorship under false pretences. The book would surely write itself. Commonwealth Fund Fellows were, by definition, highly intelligent and articulate persons. During each of the years covered by this anthology, some twenty graduates of United Kingdom universities plus five civil servants from the United Kingdom and five more from Dominion Government departments have set sail for the United States; since 1950 two Oversea (Colonial) civil servants, and since 1951 up to three editorial journalists have swelled the annual total. All these men and women were selected by a distinguished Committee of Award. To pillage the informal reports written by such post-war Fellows as these would, I thought, be no more than an agreeable spare-time occupation, and at the end an Olympus-eye view of the United States would be there for the asking. There was even the admirable precedent of the late Edward Bliss Reed's *The Commonwealth Fund Fellows and Their Impressions of America* (1932) to provide a model and obviate prefatory explanations.

But I soon found this primrose path to be strewn with difficulties. The first headache, of course, was *embarras de richesse*. Many of the reports fairly asked to be reprinted in full; others cried out for wholesale quotation—and always the editorial scissors had to keep sharp their snipping edge. Next came the vexing problem of sifting reports on specialist skills and research undertakings: there were scores of commentaries on the American

vii

academic scene, ranging from astronomy to zoology, from se-
mantics to microwave spectroscopy. I had to ask myself how
many of these records, so useful to the Fund's Division of International Fellowships in assessing the changing scope of American
university departments and thus assisting in the placement of
new generations of British Fellows, would be intelligible to a
non-specialist reader, or valuable even to specialists themselves
after a lapse of a few years. An unscientific editor, bearing in
mind the hope that this anthology may perhaps delight Dr.
Johnson's Common Reader, may be forgiven for blenching before
such a statement as this (and by a lady, too!): "Since Wino-
gradsky's vehement denunciation of the concept of pleomorphism
among the sulphur bacteria as among other forms, studies on
morphological variation have fallen into disrepute."

I must therefore apologize in advance to the Fellows who may
search these pages in vain for their masterly summary of the state
of palaeobotany or the political scene in 1948, and instead find
themselves represented, if at all, by some forgotten remark about
the Grand Canyon or a passing reference to traffic conditions.
I can only assure them that their erudition still nourishes the
judgment of the New York officers of the Division of International
Fellowships, but would require for presentation and selection
in this anthology the combined wisdom of Aristotle and Erasmus
—and to this the editor (though himself a Fellow) lays no claim.
If the editor owes a word of explanation to Fellows represented
skimpily or not at all, he must also offer special thanks to one
or two professional writers (like Marcus Cunliffe, Alex Stur-
rock, and Graeme Moodie) who have generously allowed him
to pick out plums from material they were no doubt saving for
future books.

Moreover, the reports written by the men and women appointed to the above-named five categories of Fellowships in
the Commonwealth Fund's British Program during the years
1946–1952 fell under the editor's eye one at a time and in no
special order; it was often purely by accident that one particular

comment or description came to do duty for many subsequent
rephrasings of the same observation. Indeed, the selection is no
doubt unjustly biased by an editor's natural disposition, as his
work proceeds, to take for granted certain widely held opinions
and to pounce for relief upon the statement of a minority or even
a paradoxical view. My desire to avoid an endless repetition
of the affection all Commonwealth Fund Fellows come to hold
for their "second homeland" was reinforced by two-thirds of my
professional personality. As a former Fellow, I enjoy reading
tributes to American hospitality and the human qualities of the
Fund staff; as a present Fund officer I shrink from printing them;
as an editor I find them "dog bites man" stuff. Two against one:
the Noes have it!

It seemed to me wise to allow the anthology to fall—as it very
readily did fall—into a rough pattern of four main sections, so
that complementary and even opposing views could be grouped
together as examples of individual responses to the same major
themes. (As a Fulbright professor recently remarked to an English audience: "Any generalization about the United States is true
—and so is its opposite.") Any shape this anthology may possess
is due less to the editor than to the Commonwealth Fund Division
of Publications, and the Harvard University Press, who have
strengthened the editorial hand against prolixity and the ephem-
eral. Thus buttressed, I face more calmly the authors whose
excerpts were shortened or sacrificed; thus aided, I ask the reader
to share my gratitude. I have tried, at any rate, not to weight the
scales. When the anthology began to resemble *The Encyclopaedia
Britannica* in variety of subject matter (and threatened, in the
early stages, to resemble it also in bulk), it occurred to me to
borrow another habit from that revered contemporary—the combination of impartial authority and individual scholarship represented by the use of authors' initials. If the implied responsibility
of "a Commonwealth Fund Fellow" be insufficient, a reference
to the index of contributors will serve to attribute praise or blame.

Since 1952 the Fellowship program has been extended to the

continent of Europe, and a new flavour is beginning to be noticeable in the annual reports. Since 1952, too, senior Fellowships
have been available to teaching members of the faculties of
British universities who are professionally engaged in some branch
of specifically American studies. When the time comes for a new
anthology, reports by these European and senior Fellows will
no doubt be included. At the present date it seemed unwise to
risk garnishing British fare of the 1946–1952 years with an inadequate dab of later Continental sauce or the mature spices of
"revised wisdom." The next editor will enjoy working in a roomier
kitchen.

An editor who owed less personal loyalty to the Commonwealth
Fund than the present compiler might be forgiven, even on the
basis of the inadequate and almost haphazard samples herein
represented, for expressing the view that the wisdom of the late
Mr. Edward S. Harkness in setting up the Fellowships had been
amply matched, over the years, by the judgment of the British
Committee of Award who select the lucky holders and the devotion of the Fund's officers in New York who guide their steps
in America. At the moment of writing, some seven hundred
present and former holders of these awards are scattered over
the globe. The value of their study and travel in the United
States becomes more richly apparent with the passage of every
year after their return to their native lands. They have not been
specially selected to "win friends and influence people," yet as
they grow more mature in the exercise of their professional
functions in Great Britain and elsewhere, the fact that they have
lived in the United States—have worked, laughed, and perhaps
wept there—must increasingly extend the range of the formative
pressures they are exerting, all unconsciously, on the understanding of their fellow men.

It is not for an editor of such an anthology to erect sign-posts.
But I hope that others may share my particular pleasure that at a
time when many foreign critics are sedulous to document a

"pressure to conformity" in the contemporary American scene, a group of unusually well-qualified observers should unwittingly disclose, when their chance comments are flung together in unexpected juxtaposition, a striking consciousness of that unity in variety which streaks the United States with continental contradictions and which encourages British visitors with widely differing backgrounds and interests to grope towards an individual discovery of the truth of the Union motto: *E Pluribus Unum*. Some like it. Some don't. But the wise traveller will recognize in the surface similarities of much modern American living a functional web or network lightly binding together the very real diversity of the States. As one contributor remarks: "The American people, like their land, are infinitely varied; and, like their towns, are wonderfully uniform."

One disarming quality no reader of this anthology will fail to spot: as the Commonwealth Fund Fellows have come to feel privileged to *belong* to the United States, so we feel just as free to laugh with and be critical of Americans as we feel free to laugh with and be critical of our own countrymen. It is perhaps the most striking proof that over and above all the professional and academic advantages inherent in the nature of the Commonwealth Fund Fellowships, the fortunate holders have come to treasure, as the chief reward of the foresight of the Harkness family, a shared experience of the daily American life of ordinary American families.

S. G. P.

January, 1956

Contents

II. THE REWARDS OF TRAVEL

III. ACADEMIC FIELDS AND THE UNIVERSITIES

COUSINS AND STRANGERS

The Commonwealth Fund Fellowships held by those whose comments are quoted here were awarded in the years 1946–1952. The date attached to each comment is that of the Fellow's principal residence in the United States, usually the year following award.

I. The American People

Cousins or Acquaintances?

THE FRESHLY ROLLED MAP ᕃ With the impressive commentary which could be compiled from twenty-five years of Fellowship reports it is surely significant that no *Handbook of Reactions* is provided. In this respect there is something symbolic about the freshly rolled map of the United States which is received on arrival at the New York offices. Yet there are times when the novice could welcome a "prompt from the wings": what So-and-So, engaged in similar work, found in 1934 or how Dr.— talked himself out of *that* situation in '47. Instead there is the silence of "no script provided," "no stock answers given," and for this freedom we can only be grateful, since it increases the urge to fill the silence with our answers and adds to the incentive to supply a personal script.   D. G., 1951

COUSINS AND STRANGERS (1) ᕃ Initial impressions made a sharp impact. Some of them were favourable, but there were many features of the American mode of life which aroused my annoyance. I did not immediately adapt to transatlantic life and I was dismayed at my failure to do so, for of the friendliness of my hosts there was no doubt from the start and I for my part had anticipated little difficulty in feeling at home. After a few months I realized that therein lay the reason—I had expected to "feel at

1

home" in a country in which life, though faster, would follow essentially the patterns of life in Britain. And, since I had as much nationalistic pride as most Britons, I was in this mental image paying the highest compliment to America and Americans.

It is perhaps odd that I was thus unprepared for the vision of America that ultimately greeted me. I had spoken to Americans and to people who had visited America, I had read American books and followed accounts of American happenings in the press—but somehow I had never fully believed the pictures of American life they painted. I assumed that the picture was over-drawn, with an over-emphasis on the extreme or bizarre that took them almost into the realm of myth. There were others who assured me that Americans were much like ourselves, cherishing the same ideals, nourished in the same traditions, members as it were of the same family. I preferred the latter version. Like most Britons I accepted that leadership of the world had passed to the American nation. It was a consolation to know that the torch had passed to a close family friend.

It was, therefore, a shock to discover that there were in fact marked differences in American and British patterns of life—not so marked as the movies had portrayed but nevertheless considerable. It is a measure of my British complacency and smugness that for at least two months I did not question the validity of my subconscious acceptance of Britain as the model for comparison—and found much to criticize. Americans were undoubtedly "go-getters"; but where were they going and did they want anything worth while? There was much that seemed vulgar and ostentatious, superficial and materialistic; American frankness was often plain rudeness; the police were an undig-nified bunch of thugs; the cities were creations without a soul; the radios were good but the programs were an abomination; and much more besides.

It was odd to me that, despite this dreadful environment, the Americans I met continued to be so very likeable people. And then it dawned on me that perhaps I was unjustified in accepting British ways as the basic norm of human behaviour, that this was a country with a history of its own, traditions of its own, and standards based on that history and tradition. From that time I felt at ease. I sallied forth, bought myself something bright in neckwear and socks, and enjoyed myself thereafter to the full.

J. D. R., 1951

COUSINS AND STRANGERS (2) ह੭ When I set off last October to see America for myself, it was really for me a voyage of discovery, to an Eldorado and New Found Land. I was not at all sure that I should like what I found, fearing to be driven further into rather than drawn out of my shell, to be made to feel old, tired, and effete by so much confidence, so much noise, and so much progress; having no doubt that ambivalent attitude, half envious, half scornful, which always has been and perhaps always must be present when an older culture meets a newer, when the Greek traveller first came to Rome, the Indian to London.

What did I find? First, much to admire and much to love (I have in fact been affected with a wholly unexpected nostalgia ever since I returned); secondly, that far from being driven into myself as I had feared, I felt myself drawn out, warmed, charmed, I almost said rejuvenated, by the encounter with so much vitality, so much hospitality, so much genuine warmth of feeling and by the tremendous and enviable emanation of youth and vigour which is given off even in the comparatively languorous and easy-going South; thirdly, that though much was extraordinary and therefore fascinating to me, much was extremely familiar. Half the charm of the United States to an Englishman, as I suppose half the charm of England to an American, is this double face of the cousin and stranger, symbolized most of all perhaps in the language, at once different and the same, older and newer; older in that it carries so many Elizabethan and seventeenth-century words and turns of speech long lost to daily use in England;

newer, being richly loaded with fresh words and new-coined phrases. Fourthly, and of course, I found much to criticize (as what traveller and guest does not?). Though an experienced and I hope tolerant traveller, I unexpectedly found myself (because, I think, of this same familiarity and sense of kinship) questioning, comparing, and criticizing manners, institutions and methods in a way which I do not think of doing when travelling in France or Italy. I believe this exaggerated itch to compare and contrast (instead of accepting as simply and necessarily different) afflicts the American traveller in Britain in much the same way. It is a tendency against which one must guard. It reflects good sense and proper curiosity to ask, "Why do they do it this way?" but one is less often justified in asking, "Why *don't* they do it *our* way?"   J. H.-W., 1953

ANTEDILUVIAN ᙖᎨᎹ Our English host told us of an earlier *faux pas* of his (which undoubtedly added to his popularity in the area). When he was asked at a large youth conference by a pretty young girl, "What is your dating system like in England?" he answered, "I suppose it is the same as here; you know, A.D. and B.C."
                                                           A. J. W., 1953

MODESTY ᙖᎨᎹ The Americans are such poor propagandists in their own behalf. They expect to receive the respect and gratitude of Europe, to which they are so justly entitled through their efforts in the war and in the period of reconstruction; and the reputations in Europe of Roosevelt and Marshall show how gladly due honour is accorded them. But the average man on this side of the Atlantic has his knowledge of America based largely on the productions of Hollywood, at which most reasonable Americans are inclined to laugh, and on the political scene, of which most reasonable Americans tend to feel slightly ashamed (especially in election year). If the European thinks of an American city, he will usually think of New York, which is the least representative of them all. Hollywood, politics, and New York are America's principal cultural exports, yet her worst advertisements. Only by living in the United States, travelling in it, meeting and talking to ordinary people, learning their points of view, enjoying their boundless hospitality, and seeing them at work and play amid their own surroundings, can one really begin to learn their full capacity and their full worth. Unfortunately, people usually tend to accept one at one's own valuation, and if America so consistently underrates herself in the view of herself she shows to the world her stock will never amount to very much, no matter how much money she pours into the coffers of exhausted Europe. As it is, you have to go out and find the real America, or rather, the real Virginia or New Jersey or Arizona on which to form a composite picture of the real America. It is not, perhaps, very welcome to point out that the European lack of understanding of the U.S.A. is due largely to the United States themselves, but I feel it is very true, just as it is very true that there *are* good forms of democracy which are not American. The United States have the greatest responsibility that any nation has ever had in the whole course of history. Not all Americans realize it. For a start, they should stop giving themselves and other people a false idea of the sort of people Americans are. Their Constitution is much less perfect, and they themselves much more admirable, than they ever seem able to realize.   A. G. W., 1948

"It's All True" ෴ I knew New York would be busy and frantic and hot and oppressive and magnificent, and often, as when first seen from the distance as the sun is just rising, beautiful. I knew Pennsylvania Station was like a cross between Buckingham Palace, Piccadilly Circus, and a Public Convenience. I knew that an impressive number of families had at least one car. I knew that the country had, by British standards, a colossal surplus of space. I knew that America was wealthy, as shown for example in its highways and above all in its many superb and impressive bridges. I knew too that it had poverty and slums and loathsomely ugly industrial areas. I knew it had a heterogeneous population, all of whom were yet distinctively Americans, and a so-called "Negro problem." I knew that Americans were among the friendliest and most hospitable of peoples to be found anywhere in the world. I knew its population included millionaire moguls of industry and finance, Park Avenue matrons, cracker-barrel philosophers, Helen Hokinson committee women, conspicuous consumers, religious and other cranks of all varieties, and I had even heard there were large numbers of just ordinary people. I knew there were political corruptions, and Red scares and witch-hunts, and here and there a few radicals, or even one or two Reds. I knew all this, and more besides, before I went to America. But not until I had been there did I completely believe it. "It's all true" was thus my first impression of America.   G. C. M., 1950

"YOU'RE WELCOME" ૱ Broadly, any difficulties and misunderstandings which are likely to arise between Britons and Americans would be likely to come from the similarities between us rather than our differences. The material things, such as people, language, manufactured articles, countryside, all have a superficial familiarity. One feels one could slip easily from the one life to the other, but all of these things have an irritating way of not being quite the same as they appeared at first sight. This applies equally to mental outlooks and values as to material objects. It would perhaps be better if there were some obvious indicator of a different nationality such as colour or language to warn us that America has indeed a different nationality from our own.

What was more surprising than finding how different we were was the rapidity with which the differences were dispelled. Almost before realizing that some adjustment in thought and outlook was necessary I found that I was already at home in the States. The ease with which America greets and absorbs the stranger is of course well recognized, and this open-heartedness is in the main an inborn character although much of the early schooling stresses the development of community spirit and social relationships. The "get together" spirit is continued in adult life through the medium of the various business and professional and social societies. One has a slight feeling on first acquaintance with the more official welcoming organizations that the ease and warmth of the processes of introduction are too smooth and professional to have any real meaning behind them, but on more prolonged acquaintance it appears that this warmth and pleasure are basically real with addition of a practised art of making the stranger feel at home.

The difference of response between entering a strange community in England and America is one of the most striking comparisons of the two societies—the English instinctively commencing with distrust and suspicion which is only removed by fairly long contact. The reasons for the American attitude are complex, but one of them must undoubtedly be connected with the conscious necessity of having to absorb large numbers of foreign immigrants, added to which is the survival of the "frontier hospitality" when the early settlers had constantly to depend on friends and neighbours for help and even existence. S. F. B., 1952

HOMO AMERICANUS ❧ I liked the Americans. The simple statement expresses my feelings better than a string of particulars; but if I must be specific, I found them tolerant, kindly, courteous, hospitable, easy in social relations, open and generous in temperament, full of zest and enthusiasm, and with a certain fundamental decency—I can't find a better word—an absence of pettiness and something very honest and direct in their instinctive reactions. I can still be overwhelmed in retrospect by the size and variety of the country, the statistics of population growth, of steel output or of industrial productivity, but in the last analysis I feel that the best things America produces are Americans.

My enthusiasms are not usually uncritical and I don't think I swallowed America whole. No doubt I was fortunate in the people I met; no doubt there is a sinister criminal underside to American life; no doubt there are confusions of values, political, moral, and aesthetic; no doubt the setting they have made for themselves is in many ways unworthy of a great people, their towns chaotic and unlovely, their countryside disfigured by advertisements, their natural resources abominably squandered; no doubt in many ways they are immature, impatient, avid of quick results, uncritical, apt to see things in black and white, and unaware that there are standards other than American ones. It would be easy to lengthen the indictment, and to document each count from unimpeachable American sources. But while the faults of contemporary America are in many ways those of the contemporary world, its virtues are mainly its own and I only wish that they were more widely shared. Certainly the traveller like myself has reason to be grateful for the friendliness, good temper, and real consideration with which he is treated everywhere. American hospitality is anything but the mere careless largesse that goes with abundant resources; there is much more to it than that, in the thoughtful consideration that springs from real imagination and sensitivity. I think that Americans at home are the politest people I know, with both the politeness of natural good manners and an engaging touch of formal courtesy that has something eighteenth-century and Virginian about it, like the origins of the Republic itself, like the origins of American democracy, too (or so it seems to me), which says, not "I am as good as you," but "you are as good as I," and asserts its own claims only in conceding those of others.

It may have become apparent by now that I was particularly happy in America. If I go on to add that from the first I felt at home there, I realize that I am starting a question which goes to the roots of Anglo-American relations—whether any Englishman has the *right* to feel at home in America; whether he is not thereby betraying his incomprehension of certain fundamental differences. My own evolution in this respect is probably like that of many others. I started off, I think, rather determinedly conscious of differences, reminding myself that we were separated by three thousand miles of ocean and a century and a half of history; that the United States originated in a revolt against England and, in a sense, is "anti-English" as a condition of its existence; that since the Revolution we have fought each other once, in 1812 (remembered by Americans and usually forgotten by Englishmen), and have been on the verge of war on several other occasions; that the Anglo-Saxon is now only one of many stocks in the composition of the population; that some racial groups have a fixed antipathy to us on principle; that many of our most cherished institutions are either incomprehensible or distasteful to the American mind; that to a large section of the American press and Congress we appear mainly as a nation of most deplorable habits, ranging from imperialism to trade discrimination, and from dragging America into our wars to defaulting on our debts afterwards; that in private intercourse our reserve is sometimes taken for rudeness, and our politeness for patronage; and that a common language may only increase the opportunities for dislike and misunderstanding (should we like Russia any better if we could all read *Pravda* in the original?). I measured these reflections against what I knew of Anglo-American co-operation in peace and war and the innumerable ties of private friendship between us. As an Anglo-Irishman I knew all about the complexities of *odi et amo* between two peoples that know each other only too well. It seemed best to keep the mind open; I promised myself an interesting time, and was prepared to enjoy everything as it came, while expecting it might be necessary to walk delicately on occasion.

I need not have worried. Either I had exaggerated the problem, or there was a closed season in Anglo-American hostility for the duration of my visit. My hosts treated me as one of themselves,

with the addition of just that amount of *empressement* one re-
serves for someone who has come a long way to see you, and an
unconcealed enjoyment of my exotic accent. I soon felt as though
I had lived a long time in the country. New York is comprehensible enough for anyone who knows the great cities of Europe,
and I took to it immediately, but I was made no less free of
other parts of the country; some of my pleasantest recollections
are of the most rock-ribbed Republican, isolationist and un-
English (German, Dutch, or Scandinavian) parts of the Midwest.
Under all regional differences I came to recognize *homo americanus* as an unmistakable type, but in retrospect I find myself
thinking of my American friends as simply my friends, reserving
the adjective for description rather than for division; we argued
and often disagreed but remained friends, and at the end of it
all we had I think resolved our conflicts, if not in agreement, at
least in an amused and happy comprehension of differences.

No one supposes that differences between nations can be
settled between individuals. There were in fact plenty of public
disagreements between Britain and America during my year: on
Korea, on China and the U.N., on rearmament in Europe, on the
NATO appointments, on the Spanish-American agreement, and
a dozen other matters. As a civil servant I had to avoid political
controversy, though it did not always avoid me since Americans
are interested to know about our domestic affairs and though one
can be discreet in public one cannot always evade the point entirely in private conversation. But I have no need to tread on
controversial matters here and I am concerned merely with the
general aspect of relations between the two countries; I will try
to put my personal views as succinctly as possible.

Like most of us I have my gloomy and my cheerful moments
on the subject; sometimes after reading the Hearst or Scripps-
Howard press or the *Chicago Tribune* I feel that nothing can
bridge the gulf between us; at other times, after we have worked
together all day and relaxed together in the evening it seems

ridiculous to think that there is any problem at all. My considered view however is that we are united by community of interests in the first place and by sentiment only in the second place; if I had disliked all Americans as cordially as I in fact liked them I should still wish to go on record as a convinced believer that neither country can in the long run do without the other. In the short run however it makes a great difference—and may make all the difference—whether we can eliminate friction in our working relations, and my evidence, for what it is worth, is that there are no two nations which ought to find it easier to work together; in fact, if we cannot do so, we may as well give up any ideas of international co-operation on a larger scale. That we spend so much of our time in criticizing each other is really a hopeful symptom: *Qui aime bien, châtie bien.* It is not altogether misleading to call it a family relation if one remembers the real facts of family life, the chief of which is that you are polite to the stranger but that no holds are barred when you are telling the other members what you really think of them, and if one does not expect family life to be an unbroken session of mutual admiration. Possibly indeed relations would be improved, rather than endangered, by more outspokenness on our side. But that is a delicate question, and there are too many awful examples in the past of visiting Englishmen who have felt the missionary urge to tell America just what is the matter with her. At the risk of sharing their fate I must, however, from the relative safety of these pages, balance my appreciation with a few words on the other side of the picture.

My affection for Americans does not prevent me from thinking that on public matters they are often wrong, and sometimes almost wilfully wrong. Their country is so vast that they can easily forget the existence of anything outside it, and treat America as the norm of human affairs and the rest of us as falling short of it, in our various degrees, either through plain incompetence or because we have not yet remodelled our institutions on the American pattern. They attribute to their own institutions, or to their innate virtues, an unexampled standard of living which is due largely to the bounties of nature and to the historical accident that gave a century of peaceful development. They have most of them little history and little direct acquaintance with the non-American world; their education does not help them to take the wide views, and their habit of mind is practical rather than analytical. Their admirable ethical bias sometimes blinds them to the play of non-ethical forces in the world outside, though no one knows better how they work in the world they know. They think more easily in quantitative than in qualitative terms, and have a weakness for the statistical media and the public opinion poll. They will prescribe American solutions for other people's problems even where they are unwilling to accept them for their own; thus they will urge federation on Europe but not for Central America, and preach tariff reductions to nations from behind the barriers erected by the Smoot-Hawley Act. In all this they are not so unlike the rest of us, and in particular they are more like nineteenth-century Britain than they or we always care to admit. But whereas we came to world leadership by a process of evolution extending over centuries, to the Americans it has come unsought and even unwanted, within the span of a single lifetime. Two reflections are inevitably prompted by one's first journey over the length and breadth of America; one, how American isolationism, which can seem so blind and selfish as viewed from the other side of the Atlantic, is a natural and almost a sympathetic growth in a country which, with all its energies and interests in the development of its own estate, has had little to spare for what lies outside; the other, how quickly and with, on the whole, such courage and realism, America has taken over its world responsibilities. Events have moved so rapidly that it needs a conscious effort to think back to the period of the Neutrality Act and the cash-and-carry provisions only ten years ago. . . .

It was in another crisis of Anglo-American relations that we were told that a great empire and little minds go ill together. To maintain our dealings at the level of candour and magnanimity which befits two great nations will always be a test of the generosity of our own temper no less than that of Americans; but for those of us who have had this experience of being admitted to an intimate share in America's life and thought, to fall below this level would be the unforgivable failure. It is good for us to know that America is there, and that on the whole, when all the controversial dust has settled, most Americans feel for us both friendship and esteem and want nothing more than to see us prosperous, powerful, and independent. Many have said to me (and found the word that I need above all to hear said): "We need you, no less than you need us."   A. H. M. H., 1951

L.C.D. AND H.C.F. ご In a country supplied by mass production and nurtured on mass education it is perhaps not too hard to find the lowest common denominator. To arrive at the highest common factor is more difficult.   A. A. P., 1951

NOTES ON CONFORMITY (1) ご For the first time the immensity of the continent was revealed to an imagination that could not grasp before the limitless area of the states of the interior; the shock of the succeeding cultures—the French at New Orleans, the Spanish in Texas and New Mexico and Arizona, the Indian, the Mormon, and the Chinese—at last my mind was too full to take in any more. I hope that I may regard conflicting American policies with greater tolerance, and recognize in American people those qualities of simplicity, of courage, and of a strong spirit that they still must exhibit in many parts of the country in order to sustain a way of life against unwilling nature. They may wear mail-order clothes and buy branded goods at their local stores that differ only slightly from place to place, but the difference in the peoples is the difference of European countries. They are bound by such hard-won ties, cherishing the bond because it represents an achievement of security and prosperity, that any threat to loosen it must be opposed by a violence that strikes a milder ear as brutal and an English ear as undignified and sentimental.   N. P. G., 1951

NOTES ON CONFORMITY (2) ८᠍➷ What kinds of unity are necessary in a society is an open question. But it seemed to me that nearly all the characteristic virtues of America spring from the mobile and relatively unstructured nature of society—the freedom, the zest, the ambition, and the energy which have made the country so prosperous and which make it such a refreshing place in which to live. I cannot think that the attempts now being made to impose something called "Americanism" as a standard to which all should conform could be anything short of disastrous were they to succeed, but I feel fairly confident that they will not succeed.   A. H. B., 1952

NOTES ON CONFORMITY (3) ८᠍➷ The actual conformity seems most marked among the younger generation; which, if true, probably results from the tremendous developments in communications in the last thirty years, so that the youth of all parts of the continent are much more subject now than previously to similar influences. The pressures are pervasive, and their effect can perhaps be summed up by saying that it is much more difficult in the U.S. than in Britain to be an eccentric and still maintain fairly normal social relations. This is, of course, by no means only a political phenomenon. Its extent can easily be exaggerated, as it often is. For, in fact, American society continues to throw up a fair number of "mavericks" (although often to be a maverick is to be subject to very great mental and nervous strains), while it is easy to be misled by the fact that Americans normally exhibit most openly those personal traits which they share with others rather than those which differentiate them. However, in itself this last point indicates the pressure to conform and underlines a difference between America and Britain. For in Britain a fairly common type of affectation, and even snobbery, is the emphasis, exaggeration, or invention of traits which show a person to be "different" or a "character."   G. C. M., 1950

NOTES ON CONFORMITY (4) ટ&ว Despite awareness of the immense human and geographical diversity to be found in the American scene—it would be impossible to travel more than a thousand miles in the U.S. without some such awareness—the most general and fundamental impression I have felt is that of overwhelming social pressures towards assimilation, and the liquidation of cultural and personality differences; of forces driving the individual to conform as quickly as possible to certain conventionally stereotyped patterns of dress and behaviour. Minor details differ in different regions, but there is to my mind very clearly a master pattern, or matrix of personality, which is now impressed upon all individuals male and female, young and old. This extreme process of assimilation is I think best referred to by the term "homogenization" invented (I believe) by the American dairyman or milk seller.

This process of homogenization of individuality is no doubt in part a natural consequence of the mechanization and mass-production of the means of communication and expression which affects modern man almost everywhere. But in America this tendency has reached its extreme development. The result in many cases is a morbid dread of being thought to be in any way peculiar, with a marked intolerance of eccentrics.

This hostility now shown strongly and overtly towards the eccentric and cultural nonconformist (who is now liable to be labelled a "Communist" by many others besides Senator McCarthy) marks, I believe, a vitally important break with America's past tradition of toleration, of individual differences in personal behaviour and belief, which no one in the "Atlantic Community" can afford to overlook. It would seem likely, unless checked, eventually to produce cultural sterility.

Consequently I have been tempted to wonder, perhaps rashly and even impertinently, whether these pressures towards homogenization are not now altogether too strong and pervasive for the health of the "American way of life." Speaking as an outsider I would say that one is apt to get an impression of the present immense richness and variety of human and natural resources of the U.S.A. being steadily pressurized into a uniform mixture. . . .

Unless America can, in the immediate future, develop a fundamental creativity in the field of basic ideas (as opposed to merely developing those of others by improved techniques) commensurate with its present vast richly mixed population and resources, the outlook is dark indeed. What strikes me as being a disquieting feature of the present cultural situation in the U.S.A. is that, so far from the trend being towards greater creativity, the reverse seems to be true, despite America's vast import of refugee genius and talent since the rise of totalitarianism in Europe. What native American figures has the U.S. today to equal its 19th-century Whitman, Hawthorne, Melville, and Henry James in literature; or its William James, Henry, and Gibbs in science; or its Ford and Rockefeller in business enterprise? Perhaps the answer will be that the days of such giants are over. But surely this is not good enough for a country which prides itself on preserving individual initiative. I have regretfully come to the conclusion that the fear of being "eccentric," or being "unlike the Joneses," which is so marked a feature of the present American way of life, is stifling the creativity which would otherwise now be in full flood.   H. A. C. D., 1951

Personalities

MR. PRESIDENT ࠺ Abilene is, as somebody remarked, a 110 per cent normal little midwestern farming town. One's first sight of it on the horizon is a grain elevator rising from a clump of trees. It lies far enough West to need the pleasant shade, in its residential area of white-painted frame bungalows, of these trees. Its chief building is a six-storey hotel, and the square brick stores along the main street display a variety of agricultural goods and machinery.

It is bisected by railroad tracks, and though the General's parents' home (now a local "monument") is not a log cabin, it is not only small for so large a family, and stuffily Victorian and replete with evidence of plain living and high thinking (*Elmer Gantry* was the only surprise in a bookcase of devotional books, *How to Select the Laying Hen, Uncle Tom's Cabin, The Officer's Manual,* and the collected poems of Whittier and Longfellow), but is strategically situated on the Wrong Side of the Tracks.

The mildewed prints on its walls suggested at once how far the General has travelled to be, in his spare time, a Churchillian amateur painter, and why he should be just as happy copying a grocer's calendar onto canvas if no other subject offers.

By midday on June 4, 1952, a sizeable crowd of country people from the surrounding area had parked their cars and gathered between this little house and the railroad track, encircling a small beribboned dais that had been erected on the site of the "Eisenhower Museum," the foundation stone of which the General was to lay. The train drew in promptly, and General Eisenhower stepped out, neat in his unfamiliar civilian suit and Army-issue monk's shoes, waving his arms and smiling that broad and infectious smile of his.

All the way along to the dais he was shaking hands, recognizing old friends with spontaneous gestures of pleasure. There was nothing unnatural about the crowd's reciprocal pleasure in his appearance. No wild cheering, but hand-clapping and smiles, and a buzz of approval for the returning Mr. Deeds.

It was a moving and dramatic moment, this first appearance of Mr. Eisenhower the candidate, fresh from the company of captains and kings, in the sleepy town of his boyhood (though it is true that for the townspeople themselves the whole affair was in a sense a repeat performance of an earlier "return" after the war's end). And for me at least, he proceeded to make the most moving and dramatic speech I was to hear from him throughout the campaign—without notes, on the theme of returning home, of parental love and character, of poverty and uprightness, of deep and unsophisticated religious feeling.

The General's wife and brothers sat with him on the platform, and the whole affair was genuine and "right" in scale; the scattering of TV and radio recording vans through the crowd, the tall hats of the imported Texan delegation were too unemphatic to suggest either political or publicity organization. Later, between thunder-plumps, there was a parade of home-constructed floats depicting incidents in the General's boyhood and adult career. He viewed it from the hotel balcony, waving and smiling and "mugging" quite unaffectedly, catching autograph albums slung up to him from the crowd, being nudged in the ribs by Mrs. Eisenhower as she called some person or incident to his attention.

Band after band filed past and he marked time to the marching tunes and held his hat over his heart for the colours. Riding clubs clattered by on horseback and he waved to the pretty girls. This, one felt, and surely the General felt also, was politics as it should be, cheerful and spontaneous and small-scale.

Later still, in another lull in the atrocious weather that had now blown up out of a clear sky, there was a ceremony of a different kind. The General was scheduled to make his first official speech of the campaign, over a nation-wide "hook-up," at an open-air meeting in the town park. Ten minutes before the deadline, the streets were awash with water and the park a sea of mud. But at the last moment the rain stopped and the speech was made.

It was a dull, cliché-ridden speech, delivered by a small bare-headed figure in a mackintosh buttoned to the neck, grey hairs lifted wispily by the breeze, big horn-rimmed glasses dimmed by the damp air. Against the huge grey backdrop of a thundery sky there was something Lear-like in the scene, as the General ploughed his way flatly and abruptly through the ghost-written paragraphs in a nearly empty arena, with half of his sparse audience in cars whose horns punctuated his speech with mechanical applause, and the other half, many of them barefooted in the mud, clad in the bright, bedraggled remains of their parade costumes. The flags on the platform flapped in the wind and the sound was magnified by the loudspeakers into the rumble of distant and not unapt artillery.

Next morning, in Abilene's Plaza Theatre, its walls decorated with that international brand of sleazy *art nouveau* peculiar to the cinema, General Eisenhower gave his first press conference, answering questions posed, in the main, by Washington and other national correspondents there for the occasion. A last-minute decision to televise the conference indicated one of the many paradoxical effects of this new political weapon, since for technical reasons the candidate's replies were only half audible to the theatre audience though perfectly clear to the listeners and viewers around the nation; the kleig-lights were hot and stuffy, and the timing of the affair was artificially tailored to the network's program-timing.

The unfortunate impression left by the fumbling, storm-swept set speech of the evening before was wiped out by the General's press-conference facility. Questions were answered frankly, incisively, and in what Governor Stevenson was later to describe punningly and witheringly as "General terms"—but at this state general principles were all that seemed required of the returning hero. Ignorance, where it very understandably existed, was frankly admitted. The rueful schoolboy, the simple ex-military man, the doggedly high-principled village elder all appeared in the expressions that chased one another across the General's ruddy and open countenance.

If a gap in knowledge concerning tariffs and overseas trade was a little disquieting in one so recently back himself from overseas, this on the whole was easily overlooked in the atmosphere of pleasure and satisfaction generated by the unorthodox honesty and empirical warmth of the new arrival on the political scene. The press, certainly, left the Plaza Theatre, Abilene, in a mood of glowing approval.   A. P. S., 1952

THE PRESIDENT MANQUÉ &~ I travelled round southern New England for a few days with Governor Stevenson. His speeches were intelligent and eloquent, his personality pleasing and a little remote. British reporters fell for him resoundingly—he was a breath of home to them. There was some justification of American criticism of the biased election picture presented to Europe, for too few of the visitors seemed to be able to ignore their own feelings in the matter, or to appreciate that "Englishness" or even "Frenchness" is not a quality that appeals to the American voter as much as to an Englishman or a Frenchman. This is not to say that Governor Stevenson, whatever his personal characteristics, is not—or at least was not—a major star on the political horizon. He summed up the case, and as it turned out pronounced the funeral oration, for the New Deal–Fair Deal era with an intelligence and verbal grace that were at times almost Periclean.
                    A. P. S., 1952

THE EX-PRESIDENT &~ Mr. Truman is not a great man. He is small-town, Midwest, and a professional ward politician to his finger-tips. But his choice of advisers had been far better than the mere record of cronyism would suggest. At this stage, it is difficult to see what better major decisions on international and national affairs could have been taken than those taken by him. History may prove otherwise, certainly, but in the meantime Mr. Truman's last and greatest personal decision—not to run again—seems to have been as right and as praiseworthy as most of his others.   A. P. S., 1952

Landscape with Figures

DUEL IN THE SUN ₰ I arrived in New York at the beginning of September, 1951. It seems a very long time ago. I had the sky-scrapers—"secular Gothic," I noted industriously in my new diary —and the "El," and the lights of Broadway, and my first drugstore breakfast to digest both physically and mentally, as everybody else had had to do who arrived in New York for the first time. Of all that happened in the first month one small and inconse-quential memory remains most vivid.

We were walking on Fifth Avenue, up in the 80's, beside Central Park, and the temperature was well up there, too—warm for that time of year even to New Yorkers, and to me, still in my British clothes, very hot indeed. Butlers from the grand mansions on the east side of the street were exercising poodles in the shade of the park trees. Nursemaids were escorting children in sunsuits. At ground level it was all surprisingly English (though a bygone, Barsetshire redivivus, Angela Thirkell England).

A big black limousine came up through one of the tunnels from the Park and stopped with the traffic lights against it. Be-hind was a canary-coloured taxi, which also stopped, squealing, and there stepped out from the driver's seat a simian, sweating, shouting little tub of a man in a white undervest and blue cotton slacks. He advanced to the dark limousine, and from it in turn emerged a desiccated Negro (the taxi-driver was a white man) in a neat navy-blue uniform, complete with peaked cap. Some incident had occurred, apparently farther back along the road.

The Negro retreated step by step into one arc of the cross-roads, the taximan following him shouting and gesticulating, coming closer and closer and aiming kicks at the Negro's groin with a surprisingly light-footed, almost ballet-like control of balance. By this time the Negro chauffeur too was shouting, hoarsely, while their empty cars, with engines running, stood behind the red light.

Then we saw, produced from nowhere, something white in

the Negro's hand, a little knife, a penknife, with the blade unfolded. Now, in a stately minuet reversal, it was the taxi-driver who began to retreat, the Negro chauffeur to advance, with small formal stabbing movements of the knife. Both were still shouting.

Then the traffic lights changed. The two men broke off, climbed into their cars, let in their clutches, and drove away eastwards. The footmen and nursemaids, who had showed some passing interest in the affair, returned to their charges and their poodles on the sun-dappled sidewalk. That was all.

Now I describe this, not, as might be suspected, because I wish to draw any conclusions at all from the incident, but because if I had left America again at the end of that first month, I almost certainly would have. The richness of Fifth Avenue, the heat of the sun, the unbridled passions, the Negro-white enmity, the unconcern of the sidewalk observers—it was all according to Hoyle. But in fifteen months I never saw another Negro with a knife in his hand. I saw more frame houses needing a fresh coat of paint than there are penthouses in New York. The incident lives in my mind for two reasons—it was a first impression, and it came up to preconceived notions of life in the United States. One grows out of preconceived notions, but the penalty is that second impressions are never quite so vivid.   A. P. S., 1952

PRACTICAL HOSPITALITY ≳ There was the man with whom I shared a room in South Carolina when we both got caught in a blizzard, who, before he left next morning, invited me to spend a weekend at his home in Florida—and meant it. There was the owner of Buck Rogers Trading Post, at the east end of the Grand Canyon, where I stopped for a cup of coffee, who said he did not want to sell a beautiful piece of petrified wood, which an Indian had found in the canyon on the previous day, but who, as I was leaving, thrust it into my hands and would not take a nickel for it because I came from England. There was the owner of a motel outside Corvallis in Oregon, who for the same reason invited me to have breakfast with him and his wife, as their guest, before I left next morning—and the couple who spoke to me coming out of church in Vicksburg and promptly invited me to have Sunday dinner with them. Then there was the rancher near Oxnard, in California, who is a well-known local painter of western scenes and who, when I expressed a liking for one of his paintings, insisted on giving it to me—but who later decided that that one was not good enough and so painted the whole scene again and gave me that instead.

I must not forget to mention that in Texas I was invited to visit the Midwestern University in Wichita Falls and to call on the President, who, to my amazement, presented me with an expensive pair of cowboy boots as a gift from the university. Then in Ventura, in California again, I was taken to the Rest and Aspiration Club, where all the leading citizens gather once a week and where I learned something of the way in which local affairs are conducted and experienced the good fellowship and informality that are so characteristic of the West. After my second visit there I was made a full "sitting" member.

Finally I must mention the men at the gas-stations, the men and girls in cafes, restaurants, and drugstores, the rangers in the national parks and even the people in the streets—all the ordinary people of America, who have greeted me everywhere with a cheerful smile and a friendly word and have made me feel a great sense of fellowship with them all. There are many things in the famous "American way of life" (whatever that may be!) that do not appeal to me and some of which I actively disapprove, but as far as I am concerned I place the American people second to none in their friendliness, courtesy, and generosity, and I am deeply grateful for all the kindness I have received from them.

W. G. H., 1951

AUTHORITY AND THE FRONTIER ᘐᗧ The life of the frontier bred intense self-reliance, both individual and communal. The pioneers in their small communities had to improvise all their needs and this led to a high standard of initiative. It also resulted in a tendency to care little for higher or remote authority, or for the more advanced cultural values. Education of any kind is something that has to serve the immediate ends of life. It therefore has to be made as practical as possible by continuous experiment and adaptation. These ideas are of basic and enduring importance in the American tradition. Another institution that lived on in frontier life was the old town meeting of New England. This was an assembly of every single citizen whenever anything of general purport had to be decided. Although the frontier proper has been closed now for some sixty years, the spirit of enterprise which it engendered is still alive and active. The new frontier is the use of science to improve human living. One of the main characteristics of present-day America is the ceaseless quest for new and better ways of performing every conceivable service. Another is the vigorous initiative that is still shown when the feelings of the community are aroused. The American believes in action, and a tradition of success has given him the belief that it can always be made effective.   F. P. C., 1953

CONFIDENCE ﹠ To the average American, life appears good. Around him he sees solid evidence of tremendous achievement and he feels a justifiable pride in the accomplishments of his country. There seems—and even recent world events have no more than dented the optimism of most Americans—every reason why life in the future should be even better; no limit to the benefits which machines and technology can bestow. The American economic and political systems, with their emphasis on individual privilege, initiative, and ingenuity, have been vindicated triumphantly. What the American nation has enjoyed the whole world can enjoy if it will, or so many Americans believe. With their faith in the innate goodness of man and in the power of reason they are persuaded that the human intellect can devise some international order which would arbitrate all competing interests, eliminate all conflict, and usher in an era of world-wide unbounded progress and prosperity.

This Utopian concept may not be universal among Americans, and it is not confined to citizens of that country, but it is more prevalent in America today than in most countries. There is an element of self-righteousness also, perhaps fostered by the facts of geography, which has saved the nation from a too obvious involvement in or responsibility for international strife, and by the abundance of wealth which has thwarted a too obvious display of an internal social struggle. The danger of this idealism is that it is based on a generously optimistic assessment of human nature, and disillusionment may result in cynicism or even despair. The seeds of isolationism are dormant but can be stimulated to growth by an excess of self-righteousness or an abundance of cynicism—and there is plenty of evidence of commencing cynicism among some Americans today.   J. D. R., 1951

GROWING-PAINS ?❧ It takes a very long time for any way of life to become softened, rounded, and adapted, so that the people who grow up in the society can live full and confident personal lives. The problems that one encounters are such that few people can solve them in one generation; there is a certain necessity for experience to construct a framework, a pattern of beliefs, behaviour, and conventions, which may often appear irksome or ridiculous but which nevertheless shelter the individual human being from the loneliness and uncertainty of complete personal autonomy.

I suspect that rapid change is necessarily incompatible with the full personal happiness of those who are involved in it, although they may enjoy a different sort of satisfaction. . . .

There was obviously a very great deal wrong with the state which human society had reached by, say, 1800. In the evolution of better forms of society, many different paths are going to be

tried; and, one way or another, they will be very painful for
the people who tread them. In some cases the pain will be a
result of inherent factors which cannot be eliminated and which
will lead eventually to the rejection of that particular solution.
In other cases, the pain, or the emptiness, will eventually go. I
think it is a great mistake to try to pass final judgments on societies which are undergoing rapid change and growth, be they
Russian or American.

I failed to think of satisfactory answers to questions like "Well,
and how did you like America?" or "Do you think the American
way of life is a Good Thing?" There was so much that I liked
enormously, and so many things that I felt were tragically wrong,
that the questions seemed to have little meaning. Perhaps the
more meaningful question was "Why does Capitalism work so
well in America and so indifferently everywhere else?" I think
the answer has a great deal to do with the absence in America
of any permanent complex framework of attitudes and appetites,
which allows economic development to take place against very
little internal friction, and encourages people to feel confident of
being able to do all sorts of things which in societies with a
great weight of tradition they would know beforehand were
doomed to failure.

The result is great material prosperity and an almost perfect
solution to many of the mechanical problems of life; the super-
market may be the death blow to small shop-keepers, but it
does produce an enormous variety of excellent food at cheap
prices, and for people who do not enjoy spending half their
day standing in queues, seems to be an unalloyed boon. In
virtually every situation where a service or a product is desirable, it is there—shops that are open after 6 P.M., restaurants serving breakfast twenty-four hours a day, cleaners who
will wash a shirt in five hours or press a suit in three; cheap
cars, the least expensive of which look, and probably are,
a great deal better than all but the luxury class of European

cars; competent and enthusiastic garage mechanics wherever one goes; in short, a buyer's market—and we are all buyers. And seemingly unlimited money for research—particularly medical— for people feel that if enough effort is put into solving a problem, it will be solved.

But I think the absence of a deeply rooted framework of society makes it difficult for people to lead lives in which one feels they have a deep inner confidence. This was particularly noticeable amongst people in American universities, very many of whom seem desperately unsure and weakly rooted in that world. (On the other hand, they have a much livelier appreciation of the rest of the world than one suspects most of their English counterparts possess.) And in the absence of this inner certainty about things, people's opinions, their ideas on how they should live, enjoy themselves, and appear to others, are likely to be much more labile. It is obviously very difficult to assess the real influence of the extremists of one sort or another, be they the voluble supporters of Chiang Kai-shek or of a particular kind of soap-powder. Perhaps the effect that such people have is overestimated by those who finance them. H. E. H., 1954

TUBS VERSUS SHOWERS ?⤳ Now, suppose that, instead of this early morning "in-quick and out-quicker" policy, the busy wage-earner took just that little bit longer, and lay back soaking in his tub, twiddling the soap with his toes in a relaxed sort of way and reflecting on the vanity of human endeavour, would he not acquire a new perspective, a more detached way of thinking, a mellower philosophy? Would he not cease to honk his horn at the traffic lights because they were not turning green fast enough? Would he not travel all the way by the local train instead of changing to the express at 96th Street? Would he not add years to his life and his digestion? I may add, in parenthesis, that even where bathtubs were found to exist, one could not lie full length in them. This was perhaps the cruellest blow of all.

A. G. W., 1948

PUZZLES AND PARADOXES ट॰ Much seems to have been learned. That underneath sometimes appearing to know all the answers, America has the humility and even diffidence of the youthful conscience, while underneath an outward humility Britain has the self-satisfaction of the elderly conscience. That America welcomes first and criticizes second, not, as is unfortunately the case with most countries, the reverse. That formality can be an awful waste of time and energy. That Americans are paradoxical creatures—they seem to believe strongly in education for their young while being suspicious of the curious people who purvey it! They are rugged individualists in many ways, yet at the same time are under and yield unexpectedly to the pressure to conform. Perhaps most important of all was that I lived for six months (and enjoyed each day of it) with a family holding firmly such unattractive views as that Britain is a finished nation, and that my much-admired Roosevelt should have spent the major part of his life in jail.   B. M. W. T., 1951

VIGOUR AND RESTRAINT ट॰ The question which immediately occurs to one is—why is it that a town which has not existed for very long, and therefore ought, on the face of it, to look like a new town, should exhibit all the confusion and ugliness which is scarcely equalled by European cities whose development has muddled along since the Middle Ages? On travelling west I discovered that the same question essentially could be asked about any American town with a few exceptions like San Francisco, Logan, and Salt Lake City. Given all the European examples of how a city or town ought not to develop, why is it that the Americans have allowed most of their western towns (I say western because my experience east of Chicago is very limited) to become so drab, uninteresting, and stereotyped? The attempt to answer this, I think, throws light on an American characteristic which is both strength and weakness. This characteristic might be called practical energy—a genius for working with great zeal and efficiency towards some specific goal, rather tending to neglect side issues;

and in this qualifying phrase lies the snag. In the warm summers in the middle of America people get thirsty and they need petrol for their cars—and so the core of the average western town has come to be two clusters of gas-stations joined by a string of drugstores and saloons. Timber was needed for all sorts of purposes—and so indiscriminate felling has created deserts and flood-harassed death-traps. Such examples could be multiplied, but to do so would give the impression that I had a low opinion of American intelligence. And this is by no means the case. In fact, I do not regard this as having any reflection on intelligence, certainly no adverse one. For I think such a situation is inevitably characteristic of a country which has so comparatively recently been in the pioneering stage, in the broadest sense of this term— a stage in which such unlimited scope and opportunity were available to those who had sufficient initiative. A more thoughtful and less single-minded exploitation of resources is characteristic of a nation which has reached that stage at which it realizes that its natural supplies are finite. And there is ample evidence that American thought has reached this stage. Action, however, in this as in most matters, lingers somewhat behind thought, for repairing of past damages must be combined with a change of future policy. But processes of thought and communication are so much quicker now than they were in the early development of Europe that America has reached this mature stage without having had time to lose the vigour and energy of a young nation.

A. H. W., 1951

LOWELLS ξ☙ After living near Boston for most of the year, where there are tremendous barriers of reserve and class-consciousness (officially non-existent in America), it was particularly refreshing to experience the extreme warmth and friendliness of the rest of the country. G. S. K., 1950

CABOTS, KABOTSCHNIKS ξ☙ While the Spanish were building their missions in New Mexico, the Puritans came to New England.

They held two very different views of the same God. Both spoke
of converting the heathen, but the Spaniard pursued the holy
errand with zeal and a sympathy that extended to intermarriage,
while the Puritan soon came to identify the Indians with the
Devil; "when they landed they fell upon their knees—and then
upon the aborigines." New England grew by piety and trade;
Calvinism died away but left abiding traces; handsome white
houses went up around the greens, confronting the dignified white
churches. The shot heard round the world. Unitarians, authors,
colleges. Wealth from shipping. A rich and cultivated aristocracy,
with its headquarters in Boston and sturdy outposts in the other
New England towns. Pride, prosperity, and Anglo-Saxon names.

Then began the immigrant wave, as some of New England's
wealth fell off (inland, the forests cut—the lumber boom gone
impatiently west from Maine; on the coast, the little ports dying
slowly, with the passage of the sailing-ship) and as the old stock
moved out from its stony farms into new territory (a whole island
off the Maine coast depopulated, as its farmer-inhabitants joined
the gold-rush). There came the Irish, in great numbers, settling
most thickly in and around Boston; Germans, Poles, many Italians,
Jews. Odd-sounding names on the shop-fronts, strange tongues in
the street. The rhyme had run:

> Here's to good old Boston
> The home of the bean and the cod,
> Where the Lowells speak only to Cabots
> And the Cabots speak only to God.

But not even the old names were left untouched by the new-
comers. Many immigrants soon changed their names, either for
simplicity or in order to identify themselves with native-born
Americans. One such family went so far as to change its name of
"Kabotschnik" into "Cabot." The Boston Cabots were provoked
into a lawsuit to defend their ancient name. They lost the lawsuit,
and another version of the rhyme appeared: *

*From *The Proper Bostonians,* by Cleveland Amory (New York, E. P.
Dutton & Co., 1947), p. 35. Quoted by permission.

And this is good old Boston,
The home of the bean and the cod,
Where the Lowells have no one to talk to,
'Cause the Cabots talk Yiddish, by God!

The New England scene has changed a good deal within the century. There are exquisite villages—Wiscasset in Maine, Litchfield in Connecticut, or Old Bennington in Vermont. But the quiet towns changed with the Industrial Revolution. Factories sprang up all along the coast, and up the rivers where there was water-power. Immigrants from Eastern Europe supplied labour, and—more recently—Negroes came in. Catholic churches supplemented the tall Congregational, Methodist, Unitarian and Episcopalian structures. The old cemeteries remained of course, thickly clustered with old names, lovingly tended by the Daughters of the American Revolution; but the Knights of Columbus and many another organization were on hand to guard the graves in new burial-grounds. The colleges also remained, more concentrated than anywhere else in America and still perhaps more chic—to Europeans at any rate; but their prestige began to be seriously threatened by Chicago, Madison, Berkeley, and half a dozen other universities. And—alas for the old order and the D.A.R. (a startled group of whom was addressed by one lecturer as "Fellow-Revolutionaries!")—in the year that Harry Truman beat Mr. Dewey, Yale elected a Negro as captain of its football team. In the bare valleys, softwoods descend the hillsides and overwhelm abandoned fields. In the towns, business-men will tell you that the new factories are springing up, not in this cradle of industrialism but in Texas, away west and south. The tale is of decay and change. The decay should not be exaggerated— New England is still thriving by European standards—but the change is everywhere apparent. An ancestor who took pot-shots at the redcoats is still an asset, but is he as tangible as a million dollars made out of honest hot dogs and hamburgers?

M. F. C., 1949

YOUNG MARRIEDS ‿ We stayed for three weeks in San Francisco.
Two of these three weeks were spent in East Richmond Heights,
overlooking the Bay and Mount Tamalpais. Our friends were
people of modest means, who had built their own house. This
itself made them seem of heroic proportions to me. Building a
house seemed to belong to the pioneer days—to earlier and more
rugged levels of existence. L. S. did not look at all like a pioneer.
He was—and I trust still is—a schoolmaster in his early thirties,
bespectacled, with cropped hair lending a comically Prussian air
to his long, slender figure and mild academic features. He was
an excellent violinist, a child prodigy who had been performing
in his early 'teens. He, his wife and two children had worked
upon the house during their spare time for nine months, together
with another young married couple. They had done all the elec-
trical wiring, the floor laying, the foundations. The only professional assistance had come from a plumber. After living in the
house for almost a year, the other couple migrated to New York
and left the S. couple with the whole house. It had originally
been designed with two kitchens, and separate bedrooms, with
a shared living room. The S.'s then had a choice of two kitchens,
and so on. They were a delightful couple, tremendously alive.
In a way, one was reminded of Stuart Chase's books: so optimistic, warm with enthusiasm and love of life—also Stuart
Chase's rather naive pride in being "up to the moment." This is
one thing that deeply impressed me about young Americans
(although once more I "knew" this from books). But every generalization begets an exception, if not three or four, and I can
recall young Americans who seemed afraid to be enthusiastic or
forceful. L. S. himself was angry and humiliated at having signed
the Levering "loyalty oath," against all his convictions. His situation forced one to reflect upon the state of society which had
given rise to his problem. How unjust that the honest man must
become a martyr to preserve his integrity. I have enough of
sociological bias to agree with Hoffding's dictum that the ethi-
cally obligatory must be sociologically possible.   J. F. M., 1951

WIDOWS ౭ It is, I suppose, due to hustle that so many fortunes have been made, so many digestions broken, and so many widows left to a decade or two of luxury and good works. The aged and well-preserved dowager I noted particularly as an outstanding personality in the eastern scene as I knew it, and it may well be true that "Big Business" does worry a large number of wealthy men into a premature grave. Their relicts, for such I take the majority of these good ladies to be, seem to show an amazing thirst for knowledge and an energy beyond their years. At the English-Speaking Union they would flock to the meetings with great joy; they packed the Archaeological Society; they heard about ancient Babylon and modern Cambridge with equal enthusiasm; and for any good cause they were prepared to give unstintingly of their time and money. As a class I found them wholly delightful, and I am sure that their influence is both wholesome and far-reaching. It is an influence dearly bought. A little less hustle, a little slower tempo, a few more years added to the life of the American male, are possibly to be preferred to even the most philanthropic widowhood.   A. G. W., 1948

ACCENT ON YOUTH ౭ While generalizations are always fraught with considerable speculations as to whether one's sample is really representative of the whole, my general impression was that the population is by no means mature in a sociological sense, and that the emphasis of living is placed more on the retention of youth—its ambition, idealism, and to a certain extent its irresponsibility—than the attainment of the wisdom of age. This is not a terrible indictment of the American people, but is something which I found at first rather difficult to understand and which makes the first month or so on the American continent so entirely foreign to one's established principles and beliefs.
K. L. B., 1947

SOLIDARITY ౭ A feature of the lives of young people in the States is a relatively rigid segregation of age groups. While very young, children form groups of almost equal age, united by some degree of contempt for those younger or more than a few years older, and tend to spend far the greater part of their time in such groups. It is uncommon to find children listening to the conversations of their elders, or taking much notice of advice, and it is natural, therefore, that they miss many opportunities for learning by any means but direct experience. Moreover, having thus little contact with older people who have formed standards of their own, the process of formulation of private aims and ambitions is often greatly delayed. The standards of the group are readily adopted, success being measured entirely in terms of admiration elicited from the group. Thus if the general opinion in a school is against paying much attention to study, as seems frequently to be the case, the teacher is almost helpless, and the students graduate without having acquired much learning or mental discipline. It is also unusual to find university students taking such interest in some particular branch of their studies, or in some unrelated subject, that they are willing to put in some private study, and it is almost universally believed that the only way in which anything can be found out about a subject is to take a course in it. Surprise and even horror are frequently expressed by people who find that courses in philosophy and English literature are not a compulsory part of the studies of a science student at Cambridge: "But where do you get your culture from?" one is asked.   A. J. P., 1950

MANNERS ?? It is a popular belief in England that Americans behave in a free and easy way and are more unconventional than the English. I developed doubts of the truth of this picture as my experience widened. In the matter of dress, for example, I found the convention of business dress to be as rigid in the large towns as it is in England; and in restaurants of no particular pretensions, jacketless patrons were politely presented with a jacket to wear. In Washington, a newly arrived Commander (RN) who proposed to dress for a game of hockey at the small hotel at which we were staying was told quite firmly that to walk out of the hotel in shorts simply was not done.   G. G., 1952

THE PACE (1) ટેન In Los Angeles I was made aware of the hectic pace of business life in America by my uncle, who was frequently out of the house early in the morning for a business breakfast in town and back home late after a business dinner. Later on in Chicago I saw another aspect of the same sort of thing, this time from the point of view of a small shop-keeper. A friend of ours kept a radio shop and had to keep it open daily until late in the evening, simply because all the other radio shops did. Business life thus appears to be an endless hectic race to find an ever sharper knife with which to cut competitors' throats. I do not know what the reaction of a British business man would be to American business life, but as an outsider, I cannot help feeling that such intense and unlimited competition is unhealthy, in the sense that it makes a well-balanced life, in which both work and leisure have a place, practically impossible.
                                                    A. H. W., 1951

THE PACE (2) ટેન The common American, the unknown man one meets on one's travels, has time for a chat. I recall a sun-drenched morning in winter on a wayside station of the Rock Island Railroad in Oklahoma. I spoke to a station agent loafing in the sun. "Yep," he said, "this is a morning to be settin' along-side a crick fishin' in the sun."   C. H. de C. M., 1952

THE VALUE OF GADGETS ટેન The comparison of national habits is notoriously unreliable, but we consider that the people in America work with more energy, and more purposefully, than their counterparts in Britain, and that they bring more zest to their leisure enjoyments. Furthermore they apply their intelligence much more effectively to the smoothing, reduction, and control of the administration of living. Gadgets are one obvious manifestation of this applied intelligence, but it is to be found in every sphere of activity, from the quick and easy appliance for changing tires in garages, to the clock-regulated ovens, the lay-out of factories, and the arrangement of libraries. More important than the material devices used is the habit of mind which produces them—the valuable determination to release activity from minor matters of administration to something more rewarding. Perhaps the most remarkable achievement is the reduction of the administrative labours of the housewife. The arrangement of the kitchen and the intelligent use of domestic appliances leaves the housewife enviably free to participate in numerous non-housekeeping activities. We were, incidentally, impressed by the frequency with which the freed time was given to interesting, usually social, activities. I was interested in Ohio to find that many of the housewives, through membership of the League of Women Voters, were following with full information and understanding the proposed amendments to the State Constitution. Everywhere we were aware of the un-British freedom from frustrating and wasteful preoccupation with the mere business of arranging the conditions of living.   R. V. O., 1952

CONSUMPTION UNITS ➳ Small "personal music boxes" on the counters of snack bars, which play dance music "in your immediate vicinity only" for a nickel; printed announcements of the names of the bus driver in the airport bus and of the air crew in the plane; the emphasis upon custom-made attributes in mass-produced articles; the craze for the personal touch in otherwise uniform clothes (T-shirts with Christian names stamped on them; small brooches with initials or Christian names): all of these, together with the ubiquitous use of first names or "my friend" by comparative strangers, give an impression of an attempt to give the consumer the feeling that he or she is something more than a consumption unit. J. F. M., 1951

WOMEN AND CHILDREN FIRST ᘒ I now turn gingerly to the question of the ladies. For though they are fond of denying it—and some of them do it most attractively—it is they who run America, and indeed own well over half the money in the country. Why this should be, my wife and I do not know. We have sought the answer from many people. Some say it is because the men live in a woman's world from the cradle until they leave college or home. (A much larger percentage of the teachers in the United States are women than in Britain and there is not the same tradition of boys' boarding schools and men's clubs.) Some claim that women, having been given equality as a part of the country's political philosophy, go on to prove themselves "smarter" than men in equal contest and finish by running the show! Others simply say that men prefer it that way.

Whatever the reason, it results in a femininity in the atmosphere which a visitor can almost sniff on landing and a "monstrous regiment of women" which a foreigner ignores at his peril. Ezio Pinza nearly lost a million fans when he remarked to an interviewer, "No, I have not yet trained my wife to do that."

The influence of the women is exceeded only by that of the children. Occasionally people were kind enough to have us to stay in their homes for a few days. Once we got to know them well, we would say: "It is our impression of America that the wife runs the husband and the children run them both." We then listened to the half-hearted denial of the wife and the wholehearted agreement of the husband. At about this stage the husband decided that he would show these British people who really was the boss in that particular household and for the rest of our stay he gave his astonished children such a dose of discipline as they had never had before. Our friends assured us that no harm was done: Junior is very resilient. A. A. P., 1951

Race Relations

THE COLOUR PROBLEM ೭⊷ For a long while British colonies have
been the especial target of American journalists and other travellers, who, generally after a short visit, have returned home and
written books or articles deploring the attitude of the British
colonial administrator and the white dweller towards the non-
white races. The writer's own experience, after almost a year
spent in all parts of the States, is that the attitude of the average
white American, in areas where there are any considerable numbers of non-whites, is certainly no more liberal than is the case
in the British Far Eastern colonies today, in fact often less so.
This is not said in any spirit of criticism; the fusion of different
races into one community is extremely difficult and has been
accomplished in the United States, so far as the Caucasian races
are concerned, in an amazingly successful manner without
parallel in the world.

The non-white problem, however, remains and must be
squarely faced; it is indeed amongst this section of the population
that the greatest need for housing, and particularly low-cost
housing, is apparent. The preliminary results of the 1950 Housing
Census show that 27 per cent of the homes of non-white, non-
farm families were dilapidated, as opposed to only 7 per cent
in the case of whites. In addition, 24 per cent of non-white homes
were not dilapidated but lacked running water, private toilet
or bath, and nearly 42 per cent of non-white urban dwellings
were without flush toilets as against an over-all figure for all races
of 13 per cent.

Federal laws notwithstanding, the Southern States still require
segregation, and therefore separate housing for whites and non-
whites; in fact it is the practice in certain areas to subdivide still
further and provide separate housing for continentals, Negroes,
and Latin Americans. Other states, particularly those where the
proportion of non-whites is considerably less, encourage integration, the mixing of races within a community. Some cities, for

example Baltimore, have gone far in carrying out these ideas, but in the majority of cases it has finally resolved itself into the mingling of a low proportion of whites with a non-white community and, more rarely, of a few non-whites in a white community; there are practically no instances of high degrees of integration. It may be argued that non-whites as well as whites prefer to live with their own race and do not wish to mix; this has been strongly maintained in the South, where much of the old feudal feeling still exists and there seems to be a greater measure of understanding between whites and Negroes and a greater desire to provide the latter with better housing and conditions generally, provided it is on a basis of segregation.

S. C. W., 1952

THE NEGRO PROBLEM—AN ACUTE CASE ဢ During the summer vacation, we frequently came up with the discriminations against the American Negroes. One incident is perhaps worth reporting. Whilst swimming at a public beach, we were approached by the sheriff and rather leisurely asked if we could swim and dive. We were then asked to go and assist in recovering the body of a person, either drowning or drowned (no one seemed to know) at a dam lower down the river. As we arrived, the body of a young Negro was just being taken from the river. Later we learned a little of the history of this tragedy. As a result of racial incidents, Negroes were not allowed to use the public swimming beach. Consequently, they were in the habit of swimming lower down the river, at the dam, a rather dangerous place for inexperienced swimmers, and without the protection of the life guards at the public beach. Other aspects of the tragedy set us wondering. Were the sheriff and his assistant unable to swim, so that precious time had to be wasted to round up more experienced people? And why did a private mortician's car arrive before the doctor, and ambulance and emergency services? It was distressing to be brought face to face with one of America's greatest problems in so vivid a manner.   R. B., 1947

POLES APART? ﷼ As a resident of a colony which has racial problems in a greater degree than in the States I am naturally alert to the difficulty of establishing the harmonious integration of racial groups, particularly between black and white, and while the situation in America is vastly different from our own it was a valuable experience to see what the problems were and how they were being faced. Perhaps one of the most instructive illustrations of the structure and behaviour of American society I encountered in this connection was a personal one involving the adjustments of a Polish veterinarian to the small community to which he was posted as a Meat Inspector. It was told me in different ways by different members of the community who were genuinely concerned about the outcome of the appointment but who were not personally involved. The man was middle-aged and reared in traditions of a rigidly stratified European society in which a veterinarian and also a government official had considerable rank. The slaughter-house staff would recognize this rank and behave with due deference. The carcasses and organs would be placed and moved at his convenience and his word was law. In the American slaughter-house the slaughtermen would be Joe and Bill and if the inspector wasn't able to get himself called Sam pretty quickly he would likely as not be told to get the hell out of the slaughter-house. This particular Inspector's difficulties would be increased by his poor command of English and by the slightly different methods of American slaughter-house procedure, but the prime difficulty was that of the relationship between employer and employee. In America, the employees are talked to and not talked at, and regulations are fitted into the factory routine and not imposed on them. This is a working democracy which many Europeans find novel and appealing. It works well once the mechanism is understood, and it triumphed on the slaughter-house floor—but what appealed to me most was the desire and interest of the community to ensure that the foreigner should become adopted and accepted by the rest of the staff; in fact, that he should become an American.

S. F. B., 1952

PSYCHIATRY AND THE NEGRO ﹖ During the past ten years or so various authorities have stated that from 40 to 70 per cent of patients in general practice have predominantly psychiatric problems. It has become a commonplace to hear that human neurosis is alarmingly on the increase. It is nonetheless true, and it was my impression, moreover, that psychoneurotic illnesses are commoner in Negroes than in white people. Also, these illnesses tend to be severer and more difficult to treat in the Negro. This is due, I think, to two main causes:

1. The fact that the Negro—particularly the male—has a debased concept and valuation of himself dating from the earliest years of life. Self-loathing is one of his chief characteristics and there are few available channels in his social milieu for the expression of his instinctual tensions.

2. The fact that magic and superstition continue to play a prominent part in the emotional life of the Negro today. This is illustrated in some primitive Negro attitudes towards religious experience and death.

It is difficult for the white psychotherapist to adopt the necessary attitude of friendly objectivity towards his Negro patient. The psychotherapeutic situation unhappily tends to become a microcosm of the black-white relationships existing in the American culture. Both patient and therapist bring a set of unconscious distortions into the treatment. Many Negro patients are unfortunately ignorant of the psychiatrist's function. Too often they look upon him as a witch-doctor whose magical mumbo-jumbo may merge into treachery. There is therefore a great need to educate the Negro public in this matter. Another crying need is for more Negro psychiatrists, of whom there are less than a score in the American Psychiatric Association at present. This, of course, would involve the liberalization of current attitudes regarding the admission of Negroes to the medical profession.

All this, in my opinion, would be well worth while. Most people would agree that the Negro race has not yet had a full opportunity to realize its potentialities. In recent years figures like Ralph Bunche, Marian Anderson, Paul Robeson, and Richard Wright have given a hint of the contributions which Negroes in the future may make to the sum of human happiness and culture.

A. B. S., 1951

INDIAN RELATIONS: AN ADVERSE VIEW ⁇ On the whole the white American has not treated the Indian well; what is past one may, for present purposes, leave to the past, so long as no one makes any claims that the Indians are now very well off. I was most impressed with the prosperity of the Indians I saw in Canada and the comparative poverty of those I saw in the United States. In British Columbia they seem to have been accepted into the community a great deal more. In the United States they were segregated and treated as curios of a not very wholesome variety. Someone once quoted proudly to me the huge area of the Navajo Reservation as an instance of the liberality of the American policy towards the Indians. Now, leaving aside the question of whose the land was to bestow, anyone can be generous with a tract of desert. The Jews would hardly think anyone generous who offered them the Sahara as a new Zion. How the Navajos manage to eke out any kind of existence I cannot imagine; those Indians are best off who happen to inhabit a tourist area or a place of artistic interest (e.g., Taos). It takes considerable courage and a well-sprung car to penetrate the Navajo Reservation. Some attempt is in fact being made to make known the plight of these and other tribes, which inhabit poor country and rely on the trading of their handiwork for their livelihood. Yet, even so, there was a Congressman who agreed to the inclusion of the Navajos in

the Marshall Aid Program by saying that, if they were going
to keep millions of lazy Europeans, he guessed a few thousand
lazy Indians wouldn't make much difference. The Indian problem
is less visible and less pressing than the Negro problem, but I
found that only too many people were completely unaware of
any such problem at all. Before any American presumes to
criticize British rule in Asiatic India or in Africa, he ought first
to read up about his own Indians, past and present.

A. G. W., 1948

AMERICAN INDIANS: PHILOSOPHIES OF ADMINISTRATION 〰 TWO
fundamentally different philosophies have struggled for su-
premacy in the United States Indian Administration. These are:

1. Complete assimilation: This philosophy claims that the best
course is to homogenize the Indian by making him as like an
ordinary white American as possible, imposing upon him and
his children as far as possible the same basic personality structure
as that of the majority; and then to leave him to sink or swim
in the full tide of normal American life. This philosophy is an
aspect of the general American approach to the cultural and
functional co-ordination problem posed by dependent groups
within its metropolitan borders.

2. Self-determination: This philosophy seeks to give the Indian
an altogether different relation to the white majority. It strives
to let him keep and develop as many of his peculiarly cherished
cultural characteristics and institutions as possible. Indeed, in its
most constructive form it tries to erect protective barriers to
prevent the social and economic pressures exerted by the majority
from eroding the minority group's peculiar characteristics and
institutions, and it only seeks to change those which can be shown
to be definitely inimical to health and survival.

The aim behind such self-determinative philosophy is not, of
course, merely to preserve the Indian community as a museum
case for the delectation of anthropologists and tourists. It is rather

the hope that, if these communities can be cushioned for a while longer against present homogenizing pressures, they will, of their own free choice and in their own time, successfully adopt the best features of the American way of life, while retaining their own cultural integrity. . . .

Whatever may be the value of trying to steer a middle course between these two philosophies of government of dependent groups within the United States of America, there is no doubt in my mind that the directing policy in Washington has fluctuated wildly between opposite poles; and this fluctuation has engendered a deep-seated sense of insecurity in the minds of Indian Service personnel and has caused a wide-spread loss of morale.

Many of them have now got the idea that they either should get out at once or should proceed with the rapid liquidation of their jobs. This in turn has produced a feeling of frustration and insecurity, and doubt as to the future, in the breasts of many Indians. And these feelings, shown on both sides of the administrative fence, seem to me to have reacted on the general effectiveness of the United States Indian Administration, in most of the areas I have visited. The conclusion I draw from these considerations is that the prime requirement of good administration of dependent groups is a clear apprehension, by all members of the organization, of a simple and dynamic philosophy of government, adequate to cover the underlying aims of the whole administrative effort. Such a philosophy of government the British certainly possessed in the 19th and early 20th centuries, up to World War I. It was of course the simple imperialist (some would say jingoist) faith, so well expressed by many lines of Kipling's poetry, which regarded the duty of Englishmen as primarily the need to bring law and order to the "lesser breeds without the Law"; so that the dependent peoples might be free to receive the attention of missionaries and entrepreneurs without interference from those who hated the "white devil" for his novel techniques, whether spiritual or material. Since the Kiplingesque period I venture to say no great power possessing dependencies has had such an adequate philosophy of rule, except the U.S.S.R., whose aim is totally centripetal, and whose philosophy of rule of minorities is so intensely assimilative as to amount to a belief in the duty of the metropolitan power to annihilate, by force, any tendency towards individuality or separatism, a philosophy of nihilism (rather than homogenization) which must be repugnant to any but the completely inhuman and unscrupulous.

It was very interesting to contrast the demoralization in the Bureau of Indian Affairs, and in the Federal Indian Service generally, with the high morale in the T.V.A. In the T.V.A. high morale and efficiency have been maintained throughout its relatively short life of eighteen years, despite great vicissitudes external and internal. In my view this maintenance of morale has been due largely to the clear and consistent development by the T.V.A. directorate of a policy comprising both the factors I have been stressing: clear expression of fundamental aims, and a philosophy of administration imbuing personnel of all echelons with a strong sense of unified purpose and direction.

H. A. C. D., 1951

E Pluribus Unum

UNITY AND DIVERSITY (1) ⪧ The making of America was not an easy task. It was not an easy continent, from the very beginning. A shipload of settlers who landed on the Virginia coast in the 1640's had to eat one another's flesh; so did some of the Donner Party on the way to California, two centuries later. The winters were cruel, the summers stifling. The enormity of the continent can strike dismay in the traveller even today; and even today blizzards, drought, floods, and hurricanes are not rare. (In spite of what San Franciscans like to think, earthquakes are not impossible.) Even now, man's hold upon the continent is weak. Turn your car off a main road in Arizona, and if you have

a breakdown you will soon discover that civilization has no
dominance. If an airliner crashes, it may take days to locate.
And where would California be if somehow the supply of water
for irrigation failed? Its greenness would shrivel in a few days.

Only big forces could have shaped America. But these forces
were diverse, often hostile to one another. The Southern slav-
ocracy, and later the midwestern farmers, pulled against the
northeastern capitalists, the other pioneers hated the Mormons,
the cattlemen fought the farmers, the "robber barons" conducted
savage monopolistic warfare against one another, the Protestants
disliked the Catholics, the older immigrants despised the new. . . .
Why did the nation not shake to pieces under so many strains?
Partly it was a matter of luck, once it had achieved independence.
Europe was so engrossed and crippled by wars and upheavals
that the United States was able to turn Europe's distress to her
own advantage and secure prodigious territories with amazing
ease. Its neighbors were too weak to be dangerous. As far as
a title to land went—which was not the same thing as settlement
—the United States got the biggest bargains in history. Then
again, there was plenty of room for everybody for a hundred and
fifty years; America could take as many as chose to come. It was
lucky in natural resources; forests, rich soil, gold, iron, were all
to be found in abundance. And geography helped; after the
Appalachians had been crossed, there was good going by land
all the way to the end of the tree-line, in the Rocky Mountain
rain-shadow. The central river-system and the Great Lakes helped
movement. Above all, America had the dynamic idea of democracy, to ennoble what otherwise might have seemed nothing
better than a mad scramble for loot. Making America has been,
in one sense, a gigantic job of salesmanship; the appeal has been
to the flag, to the splendour (and not the loneliness) of size and
open spaces. It had to be drawn larger than life, taking Paul
Bunyans and not Robin Hoods for its folk-heroes; and for a
definition, "Why, sir, on the north we are bounded by the Aurora

Borealis, on the east . . . by the rising sun, on the south . . . by
the procession of the Equinoxes, and on the west by the Day of
Judgement." There were many failures, of course; but, signifi-
cantly, as Alfred Kazin has pointed out, it was not until the
frontier had long passed and the depression of the 1930's arrived
that Americans turned to examine "the forgotten stories of all
those who . . . had not risen on the steps of the American dream
from work bench to Wall Street, but had built a town where the
railroad would never pass, gambled on coal deposits where
there was no coal, risked their careers for oil where there was
no oil: all the small-town financiers who guessed wrong, all
those who groped towards riches that never came."[*] America
held together because there were in fact more successes than
failures; for salesmanship must have a core of truth if it is to
make any permanent gains: the colony in Greenland perished
even though the name belied the bleakness of the Arctic.

And America held together through a deliberate and incessant
effort to make it hold. The American gospel of self-help, hard
work, success, tomorrow, was preached *ad nauseam*. The creation
of national sentiment was an extraordinarily self-conscious affair,
as it must be; human beings are not altered as easily as inorganic
matter, in spite of the metaphor of the melting-pot. The immigrant's task, whether he be from Ireland, Germany, England, or
Italy, was to proclaim and prove himself an American. His duty
and his anxiety were to *conform*, which involved turning his back
upon Europe and learning English. Often the task was too difficult for the first generation, in whom old ways lay deep. The
expression of an aggressive Americanism (a Nativism, as it is
sometimes called), is to be found in the second generation, the
children born in America, indoctrinated in American schools,
who come into pathetic conflict with their parents in their desire
to be "good Americans." So anxious were immigrants to be

[*]Alfred Kazin, *On Native Grounds* (New York, Harcourt, Brace and Co.
Copyright, 1942). Quoted by permission of the publishers.

accepted that they were almost always conservative in politics—until recent years, at any rate—because however uncertain they might be as to what precisely constituted a Good American, they knew that it did not consist in criticizing one's new country. Thus the Germans and Scandinavians of the Midwest were opposed to the Granges and the Populist Party although these spoke up for the farmers' interests.

Nor was it only the recently arrived who felt the pressure to conform. It was apparent, and still is, all through American life. The teen-ager, no less than the elderly business-man, must obey unwritten but well-understood rules of dress, behaviour, conversation, and so on. Here lies the paradox that a nation of individualists is also a nation of conformists. Eccentricity is a luxury of countries such as England, which have been long formed, a luxury that countries in the making cannot afford. In them, the prime obligation is to make oneself understood, to be accepted; hence the importance of conformity to agreed standards, as of designing towns so that the newcomer can find his way without difficulty. The "100 per-cent Americanism" to which public figures frequently refer does not exist; yet they are right, for the important thing is to assume that it does. Thinking makes it so. The search is for the common ground. In American politics, therefore, we so often find that the opposing parties in an election, however violently they abuse one another, have in fact platforms that differ very little.

Nativism has uglier aspects. It has led the Americans at times to persecute the non-conformist, the man who on grounds of opinion, creed, or colour seems "un-American." Usually, such people have been tolerated; it is only at times of national crisis that nativism has shown itself. The Know-Nothings of the 1850's arose when the Union was threatened by Civil War, the California Workingman's Party of the 1870's after the panic of 1873 and the exhaustion of the mining frontier, the Ku-Klux-Klan of the 1920's after post-war troubles. At such moments unity in a huge and disparate country can only be found at the expense of some scapegoat, or *Gegenidee*. Whoever threatens "Americanism," or is thought to, is attacked. Here is a second apparent paradox: that the most confident nation in the world gives signs, at certain periods, of having no confidence. The explanation has been indicated; it lies in an ancient yet still powerful term of disunity, which John Adams expressed as early as 1796: ". . . There is no one article of my political creed more clearly demonstrated to my mind than this, that we shall proceed with gigantic strides to honor and consideration, and national greatness, if the union is preserved; but that if it is once broken, we shall soon divide into a parcel of petty tribes at perpetual war with one another. . . ."

The strength of anti-Communist sentiment apparent in the Dies and Un-American Activities Committees is comprehensible only in terms of this old fear that things may fall apart. America is still in the making and still vulnerable; national pride still needs to be expressed: such are the unspoken convictions of many. It is expressed in symbols like the Freedom Train and saluting the flag in school. Indeed, all over the United States far more national flags are flown than you would ever see in England. A foreigner who wishes to think so could point to such aspects of American nationalism to prove that it was raw, even aggressive. He would be wrong: it is new but it is nativistic, defensive.

How strong is American unity, and how potent the centripetal forces? It is difficult to answer. Geoffrey Gorer has remarked that you can follow the adventures of newspaper cartoon-strip heroes all the way across America, in correct sequence, although news of nation-wide importance is not always given adequate expression. You can also hear the same Hit-Parade tunes played on juke-boxes in all the different states, and see the same movies or buy the same best-sellers, without feeling that such cultural unity is very significant. There are undoubtedly great diversities of outlook; how much common agricultural solidarity can there be between the Virginia tobacco-planter, the Kansas wheat-grower, the Louisiana sugarcane-farmer, and the Californian with his citrus orchards? There are strenuous local prides; there is continual insistence upon States' rights. I had always thought of the *New Yorker* as an American version of *Punch,* yet the bookstalls have never heard of the *New Yorker* when you have driven west for a couple of days. You can buy the *New York Times* if you are lucky, but it will be an old copy; every town has its own newspapers. New York is still the principal cultural centre of the United States, but it is not the only one. Each large city is proud and autonomous in spirit, with its own aristocracy. The eastern seaboard is remote in thought as in distance from the Pacific Coast; the clothing styles are not quite the same; and they classify beer from St. Louis as eastern, although St. Louis is the West to many easterners. Each region puts out its own literary magazines, its own historical periodicals, and so on. Some speak of themselves as empires—the Redwood Empire, the Rocky Mountain Empire.

Even so, on the whole the United States would seem to be remarkably unified. "Empire" is a good publicity word. Dialects don't vary so much that it is a problem to make oneself understood in other areas. The telephone, the railroad, the aeroplane, the automobile draw the States together. It is true that there is no one city that leads the nation, as Paris does France; nor is there in Switzerland, which gets along well enough. Nationality groups appear to have merged with the rest of the community to a considerable degree; at a quick glance a town like Holland, Michigan, which was settled by the Dutch, is indistinguishable from any other midwestern place, except for Dutch names on the shopfronts. National cultural traits have by and large been pooled rather than preserved in any one district. Spaghetti and the hamburger are universal. The similarities (suspicion of Washington, belief in private enterprise and the American way of life) are greater than the differences. Only the South, with a common attitude towards the Negro and its lost war, seems to be classifiable as a "region" standing somewhat apart from the rest of America; and even in its case it is impossible to define its boundaries with any precision. With the exception of the South, which is changing, there is no political party based on region. America is a nation, in spite of the fact that some of its citizens speak its language brokenly or not at all. M. F. C., 1949

UNITY AND DIVERSITY (2) ᘒᔊ The American people, like their land, are infinitely varied; and, like their towns, are wonderfully uniform.   J. A. C. R., 1950

UNITY AND DIVERSITY (3) ᘒᔊ I have rashly made some sweeping generalizations. But, after all, the most remarkable fact about America is its diversity. It is from this diversity that the greatness of the nation probably springs, and it is the triumph of America that in the midst of such diversity there is also unity.
                                              J. D. R., 1951

II. The Rewards of Travel

Musings and Methods

TWIGS ON A STREAM IN ZION ເ≫ One afternoon in July I sat down by a stream in Zion National Park and gave way to despair. There were three of us; we had already zigzagged several thousand miles westward across America, yet covered only a third of our itinerary. The erratic red line of our route ran on remorselessly, through page after page of one of those handsome map-books that the oil companies will send to you, free of charge. When it first arrived it had delighted us. It had appeared to me as a sort of complimentary ticket to a continent. But now it was more like a diabolical contract from which there was no release.

These were the thoughts that ran through my mind in Zion. Zion was a national wonder, I told myself, gazing up at its sheer, gleaming walls (like so many places in the arid regions of America, Zion has an odd air of newness, like a building just opened: no soot on the walls, and still an unexpected sight in a dull neighborhood); a natural wonder, I told myself solemnly. But the sun struck down off the shining rock, and it felt more like a natural oven, even though we had found the coolest possible crevice, on a boulder jutting out over a swift stream. For the time being, I had had enough; I was quite saturated with scenery and distance; was a small blotter in a sea of ink.

There was too much of America. It was like a Lord Mayor's

Procession planned too lavishly, that began in splendour but went on too long, included too many diverse elements, and so began to bore long before it was over, because the organizers had not known where to stop. The same fault so often marred the American film or novel. How could Cecil B. DeMille or Thomas Wolfe be otherwise when nature itself overdid things? There were, it seemed to me, three possible approaches to an understanding of America. The first was to isolate some aspect of it—its political structure, for example. That was a useful idea, but it had been done before, and most competently. English people could grasp constitutional problems without ever visiting the United States; indeed, every European magazine one looked at carried articles on American politics. The second solution was a quick nibble at the fringes of the country, long enough to bite off a few impressions but not long enough to become bewildered. This attack had obvious advantages; a week in New York or Hollywood was long enough to collect sufficient material for several witty contributions to periodicals at home. Out of it came the smart generalization ("bright lights, dim thinking, quick drinks and adolescent sex," etc.) and the cocktail party anecdote. But even if I had wanted to achieve such divine simplicity, I had already seen too much to attempt it. The third approach was more honest, yet not completely satisfactory. It was to seize hold of what professors like to call the "totality"—to apprehend America in giant terms, by writing on a giant scale, by amassing detail, heaping up Whitmanesque catalogues; to cover every corner from Washington to Florida, from California to Maine. If only one put in enough, the whole might somehow prove not only to be greater than the parts, but their perfect integration. Such a hope lies behind the quest for the Great American Novel, the Holy Grail which so many novelists have sought. Wolfe was one, searching for "the great forgotten language, the lost lane-end into heaven, a stone, a leaf, an unfound door."* But there is

---

*Thomas Wolfe, *Look Homeward, Angel* (New York, Charles Scribner's Sons, 1929). Quoted by permission of the publishers.

no door to find, no one theme to unify the whole; only abstractions: "Americanism." What is Americanism? A word for public speeches. The abstractions are needed but dissolve away when they are examined.

So my thoughts went. I was lost in detail. A large painting needs to be examined at a distance, and I had my nose up against the canvas. Was not W.'s the most sensible reaction to such a situation? He had stretched flat out on our boulder, breathing heavily in something between a sigh and a snore: asleep. R. and I remained awake, however, hypnotized by the afternoon. The only sound was the endless sound of the brown stream-water, pouring down between rocks and jammed logs a few feet below us. Moving water will bear a great deal of scrutiny and any amount of speculation. So many different sources have contributed to swell its downward urge. . . . Tags came into my mind. . . . No one can cross the same river twice. . . . The gone waters and the going. . . . The men of today are not the men of yesterday. . . .

We began to throw twigs into the current, to see which would be the first to disappear round the lower bend. Soon we discovered that though the stream was swift, it was also subtle. One twig that fell favourably would be borne away on a strong impulse, to whirl downstream and out of sight; while another that fell only a little differently, might be drawn away by complex eddies, making little headway, until reaching a resting-place in the shelter of bank or boulder.

As we played this childish game, I began to recapture the lost thread of understanding. You need quiet interludes in America, among small objects, to restore proportion and escape the nightmare sense of enlargement. Here on our rock was such a place, where it was possible to see America in microcosm, and reduce the chaos to elementary analogies. There was no one theme but that was not to say there were no *themes*. Themes in abundance clustered about the central notion of Americanism, like the fasces round the ax. The stream, and the debris we threw upon its surface, would do as well as any other analogy in the necessary task of over-simplification. Thus: the blind gravitational force of water; the movement of Europe into a new continent. Europe bursting out under all kinds of tensions and energies; America receiving them, shaped by forces within the main gravitational pull. Twigs on a stream, some going fast, others settling in backwaters. Men in America, some plunging deep into the continent, others pausing in certain shallows and undisturbed places—the little inland townships of New England, the farms of Pennsylvania, the hillbilly nooks among the mountains, the pockets of strange tranquillity in the South. Even the backwaters, though, are not permanent; any flood high enough will wash them out and pour in new material—Irish Mayor Curley in Boston, Italian Mayor Celentano in New Haven, a New-World Birmingham in Alabama. . . . What forces had peopled a continent? Religion—

> What should we do but sing His praise
> Who brought us through the wat'ry maze
> To a land as yet unknown
> And yet far kinder than our own?

Land-hunger. Gold-fever. So many drives.

The stream showed them all in miniature. Of course it was much too neat a picture; the Force of Gravity–Manifest Destiny equation comes too pat. But I was grateful for any idea. At a time when I was wondering why I had come, it was natural to consider what motives had impelled all the others, for whom the journey was no tourist-whirl but a matter of life and death. What on earth had brought Nephi Johnson, the Mormon Scout who discovered the canyon in which we were resting? Only some powerful force, for whatever the easy progress of a twig on a stream might suggest, and however fashionable it is to write history in terms of inexorable movements, the settlers had not glided across the continent in any predetermined swoon. However rosy the prospectuses, the reality had been hard on the individual and his family. And the analogy of the stream did raise other questions. Where was the water going? What was the purpose of such rage for movement? What happened when, somewhere lower down, the water had no more impulse for movement?

If one were to write about America, briefly and impressionistically, the only way was to fasten upon some central theme and illustrate it with a few examples—bearing always in mind the inadequacy of any tidy notion of that sort, in a country with almost every variety of climate and race, and every standard of living from abject poverty in a desert to vast wealth in a metropolis. It seemed to me impossible to discuss the present-day United States without conveying some idea of elements that formed it, and of size and range and complication.

So much appeared to be made clear in Zion.

M. F. C., 1949

IN PRAISE OF THE AUTOMOBILE &• I have no hesitation in declaring that the only successful manner in which the continent of the United States can be seen and appreciated is by automobile. The advantages of freedom of movement, timing, transportation of personal effects and the readiness with which one can change from camper to city slicker (as the need arises) more than compensate for the disadvantages of long days of driving, temporary lack of amenities, and not infrequently, tragedies of the type covered by insurance.

In no other manner is access to the grass-roots of American life so closely and easily achieved. To know America it is not sufficient to list the names of all the cities or national parks one has visited. The essential thing is to join the flow of travellers as they cross the continent in every direction, to respond to the simple, generous emotion which follows from the sight of a registration plate of one's own state—by the honking of horns or the exchange of gossip, strangers welded by common pursuits to the renewal of an age-old relationship between travellers— to sleep under the stars in the Arizona desert, to awaken at dawn in the plains of Nebraska and follow the sun westwards day after day, or even persist in the belief that one's car is a pack-mule in order to reach some otherwise inaccessible canyon or ancient Indian pueblo.   A. B. D., 1947

CAR FOR FOUR, BEDS FOR TWO ཀ Travelling with two couples in the car made it reasonably cheap and not unreasonably un-comfortable. We found that it was possible to save money by taking turns to sleep in the car, and after a few experiments this proved successful and comfortable. We found that with a two-door Chevrolet—and no doubt with other two-door cars—the back of the front seats can be taken off by unscrewing one nut and bolt and by withdrawing two split-pins. When the backs were off, the cushion of the front seat was moved to a position adjoining that of the rear seat. A little packing was necessary to make them level. The backs of the front seats were then placed horizontally in the front of the car, stretching to the pedals. This made a perfectly good six-foot bed, and with a sleeping bag or sheets and blanket it was very satisfactory. The couple who were not using the car booked a room at a motel which we all used for washing and dressing. There was there-fore no washing from old tins, shaving in cold water, and no necessity to carry a tent, and no-one got wet if it rained. We also carried a gasoline stove which we strongly recommend; this saved considerable expense in restaurant meals, and made it possible to enjoy meals at pleasant places in the country.   R. H. M., 1952

TOO COMFORTABLE? ཀ My only regret is that travel is made too comfortable and too rapid. Insulated from the outside world by air-conditioning and soundproofing, the journeys lack the little unimportant memories and associations that mark one's travels

—like the smell of fresh rain on a dirt road and the sight and song of the different birds. I feel that even Americans are losing their sense of contact with the country through the ease and speed with which they travel over the great wide highways. It is, of course, the existence of such enormous areas of similar scenery which would make the simple and slower forms of travel, such as walking or cycling, monotonous and unattractive, but even in the more varied country of the eastern States I saw little evidence of organizations such as the Youth Hostel Association in Great Britain and similar organizations in Europe, which encourage and provide facilities for simple travel.   S. F. B., 1952

ROADS ટે People are so concerned to see what is around them that perhaps they do not pay much attention to the road along which they are driving. Some of these roads are incredible feats of engineering, and are no less incredible miracles of maintenance. Over the mountains and the deserts they go, yet no place is too inaccessible, too hot, too parched, or too steep for the highway authority to keep the surface good and the dangers marked. Sometimes, where a stretch of road was less good than usual, or was under construction, one heard grumbles from American tourists, and on such occasions felt like reminding them how wonderful it was to have a road there at all, and how pleased they ought to be that the highway authority was concerning itself with the upkeep of it even in the remotest places. The men who built the road, say, from Las Vegas to Tonopah are to my mind far more entitled to the universal veneration than General Custer, whose "Last Stand" figures so largely in bar-rooms and barber shops.   A. G. W., 1948

IN DEFENCE OF GENERALIZATIONS ટે The two-way process of impression and expression never ceases, though it is less active when one is static than during the period of travel. On many occasions I found myself thinking how infinitesimal I was in this vast universe. During my travels I entered many strange cities, quite unknown and certainly unnoticed by the people as they hurried about their very personal business of the day. Poor, disillusioned people I found myself saying. You are but a few of the millions of people I have seen throughout the country and the billions I have never seen throughout the world. No one knows you any more than you know me, yet you eat, sleep, work, and procreate, are subject to the vast range of human emotions, of love and hate, ambition and despair, are motivated by the necessity to live just as all the other people on this earth. Yet why do you care, why do you respond to the communities you have never seen and are never likely to see?

The miracle, for miracle it is, is that people do care, as only the traveller who moves rapidly from place to place is able to appreciate—whenever he pauses to contemplate these things. It is shown by the manner in which he is received as soon as he identifies himself with a member of the community, explains his purpose, and gives as equally as he receives of the spirit of human feeling. This happened to me wherever I stopped in the 40,000 miles of travelling through forty-four of the forty-eight States, whether in the sophisticated atmosphere of Cambridge or the backwoods of Arkansas, the humid bayou country fringing the Gulf of Mexico or in the still pine forests of Oregon. I was humbled in spirit by this expression of unity throughout the diverse regions which embrace the forty-eight States in the Union. In contrast with this response there were occasions when I felt intensely repelled by the monotony and crudity of "Main Street." The standardized restaurant complete with juke box, the litter of neon signs and gas stations desecrating the approaches to every city, town, and village, the profusion of overhead cables and telegraph wires which speak of a new or a relatively new community, all tend to depress the observer with their jarring, garish monotony.

So in a fit of irritation one is tempted to remark, "Oh, all

American cities are alike"—a generalization which holds no more truth than any other sweeping statement.

In a country as large as this there is, however, a place for generalizations, if only to serve as the basis for further exploration and understanding. One cannot comprehend this vast, complex social, economic and physical structure without first developing the framework of a relationship of which the details, by their overwhelming range, remain beyond the fringes of comprehension for a considerable time and in certain circumstances quite out of focus. It is only by making use of this technique that I achieved an understanding of America.

As a Commonwealth Fund Fellow I enjoyed the unparalleled privilege of extensive travel in order to observe the influence of environment upon character. As an architect I am fortunate among the professions for having been trained to appreciate the forces and aspirations which a community seeks to express in its buildings. The development of entire cities, the street architecture, and the individual buildings assume personality and character expressive of the inhabitants past and present. I was made conscious of civic pride by the public buildings, factories, parks, and communications, just as I was made conscious of the social and economic difficulties by the presence of ghettos and slum areas or, again, of the cultural activities by the profusion (or otherwise) of museums, concert halls, pseudo-gothic campuses, and solaria. The range is endless.

The close contact with the people which the Fellowship permits provides another field of fruitful research. It gave me time to learn the "how" and the "why" of such phenomena as high-pressure advertising in press and radio, regional and local variations in education, contemporary religious practices, the forces which generate both supreme confidence and insecurity at one and the same time, politics and pressure groups, the preference for tangible results and demonstrable principles evident, for example, in the faith expressed in the Constitution.

After long association I learned to appreciate the causes of these outward expressions of the American way of life; sometimes to support, sometimes to deplore, yet always to understand, acknowledge, and respect as part of the American scene.

A. B. D., 1947

THE AMERICAN EPIC ᗒ What does it mean to discover America? It may mean different things to different people, but for me it was like listening to an epic—an epic of man, nature, and history. No epic of classical times was ever worked out against such a background of vastness, space, and majesty. No heroes ever struggled against such terrific odds, or gave so much in the fight, as the countless unknown settlers and pioneers who crossed from East to West and brought this continent to habitable terms. All this is woven into the history of America, along with that other struggle of North and South. And yet how much there is which seems to be waiting for history to begin. Travel across the Mohave Desert or walk down into the Grand Canyon and it is hard to escape the feeling that you are back at the beginning of time and the only realities are the red rocks and the harsh brilliance of the sun. It was at such moments that I told myself: "If the Americans are not religious, they should be. Despite their many achievements, there is enough here to save them from pride and to remind them of man's littleness before the mystery of the world."

D. G., 1951

PLACE NAMES ᗒ For those who know how to read them, maps speak volumes. All a nation's history is to be discerned in a good map and especially in the names upon the map. The names on the American map disclose the mingled pedigrees of the nation. Naming was until recently one of the great American sports; indeed a necessity as well as a hobby, with so many new rivers, mountains, lakes, fords, homesteads, settlements, all crying out for a label. For man is a name-giving animal; as "what shall we

call it?" is one of the first questions debated about a newborn
child, so is it with any new thing. And as few men are poets,
the names given to the American scene were not always original
or euphonious. The first settlers often took Indian names for
rivers and hills—Connecticut, Megunticook—and bestowed English names upon their towns—Stamford, Portsmouth. So, on the
vast map of America we find names the Indians used and the
English brought; names the Spanish conferred—San Diego and
Santa Fe, El Paso and Albuquerque; names the French left—
Detroit, St. Louis, Vincennes, Baton Rouge; names that came
in with the classical revival—Memphis, Cairo, Rome, Carthage,
and Ithaca; names given in memory of famous men—there are
dozens of Washingtons, Franklins, Jeffersons, Lincolns. There
are names culled out of literature and many from the Bible.
There are names taken westward in the mental baggage of the
settlers—Boylston, Beverly, Roxboro, Malden, and Taunton, in
the state of Washington, were all called after towns in Massachusetts. There are genteel eastern names like Rosedale and
Cedarhurst, and the robust western ones—Wild Horse, Cripple
Creek, Bigtimber, Troublesome. There are plain, uncompromis-
ing names, like Granite and Cement in Oklahoma, or Chloride in
Nevada. There are names corrupted: thus the Spanish "El Rio
de las Animas Perdidas en Purgatorio"—a place where some early
Spaniards killed one another and died unshriven—became "Purga-
toire" to French trappers, and in turn "Picketwire." Many re-
sounding or enticing names were given to new settlements in
the optimistic hope that they would someday earn the importance
such names hinted at. There are names such as Minneapolis in
which Indian and classical roots are mated with a fine disregard
for the niceties of etymology. And there are endless examples
of places named by tacking a -ville or a -burg onto a surname.

How Matthew Arnold winced at the marvellous mixture that
resulted! "The mere nomenclature of the country," he wrote,
"acts upon a cultivated person like the incessant pricking of

pins. What person in whom the sense for beauty and fitness was quick could have invented, or could tolerate, the hideous names ending in *ville*, the Briggsvilles, Higginsvilles, Jacksonvilles rife from Maine to Florida; the jumble of unnatural and inappropriate names everywhere?" Matthew Arnold came from a country where the Scholar Gipsy might still haunt the villages around his ancient Oxford, and where a gentleman could quote the classics in Parliament and be understood. Briggsville sounded far less beautiful than Bablock Hythe, and to find a Rome and Carthage in New York State was an affront. The charge of ugliness was more valid than of unnaturalness. Briggsville, and all the other names are unimaginative. But what *was* "natural" to America? What else but a mélange of names from all over the world? As Stephen Benét says of America,*

> They tried to fit you with an English song
> And clip your speech into the English tale
> But, even from the first, the words went wrong,
> The catbird pecked away the nightingale.

The nightingale sang perhaps at Stanton Harcourt and Kingston Bagpuize; in America it was different. There was beauty of another kind to be sought there. The names on its map are sometimes dull or bizarre, sometimes lovely, in a fortuitous way, like the patterns in a kaleidoscope. But harsh or sweet, they tell the story of America as vividly as any book. They show lines of force, as iron filings show the shapes of a magnetic field, but humanize them.   M. F. C., 1949

MAN AND NATURE ᙖ Everywhere in southwestern U.S.A. I was astonished by the success of American farmers in rearing thrifty Hereford cattle on a seemingly waterless desert. This is an object-lesson for other parts of the world. In its own way, the

---

*"John Brown's Body." From *Selected Works of Stephen Vincent Benét* (Rinehart & Co., Inc. Copyright 1927, 1928 by Stephen Vincent Benét). Quoted by permission.

man-made fertility of California is of course just as astonishing;
but in and around Los Angeles especially I could not get away
from the feeling that unless the effort and the economic situation
are maintained, this whole burgeoning civilization might suddenly collapse into unpeopled desert again. The relation of man
to nature, which always in America seemed to me quite a different one from that which we know in rural Europe and the British
Isles, is of an urgent, violent kind; either man wins, or nature
does, but the partnership of the two is not a peaceable, permanent
thing, ruled as it were by natural laws. This impression I gained
no less in the Middle West and the upper Missouri Valley
(where the pros and cons of the great development scheme interested me greatly) than in California. Just as the relations between
man and nature itself are not static or stable in America, so it
seems to me that human nature itself is not static or stable, to
the American way of thinking. Perhaps this is one of the many
reasons why Americans throw so much emphasis on the American way of life, as a guarantee of consistency in a world where
everything can change, and where it is now realized that things
do not always change for the better.   R. A. S. B., 1953

TRAVEL IS PEOPLE ॐ The complexity of the problems came more
fully to our appreciation along with the experience (as distinct
from the distant knowledge) of the heterogeneity of the American people and the variety of the regions. It was the people
rather than the geography which brought home the regionalism.
The difference in mode of life, behaviour, and traditions struck
us more forcibly than the difference in countryside and environment, though related to it. Our indefinite awareness of a factor
in American life was changed, by travel, into a concrete experience. The South Carolina comment on the Sherman Central Park
statue—"Only a Yankee would let the lady walk"—and a warning
against barbarous Georgian practices in preparing mint julep
bring to mind the whole context of differing histories and customs

only half-sensed before when reading, say, Henry James' *The Bostonians*. This on-the-spot sense of the regionalism paves the way for further appreciation of American life and literature, and in itself is ample reward for the Grand Tour mileage.

R. V. O., 1952

SPACE ᢒᢌ The geopoliticians described the standard European concept as one of "Kirchturmschatten-Beschraenktheit" or the village pump spirit. To drive fifty miles to dinner, or eighty miles for half an hour's discussion, as I have frequently done in the past two years, is unthinkable anywhere else than in North America. The result is an extraordinary contraction of space and an equally remarkable broadening of horizon. This feature of American life has been frequently pointed out; I myself was skeptical until I met a Texan who twice weekly drove 120 miles to take a girl to the cinema, returning the same evening.

J. H. P., 1950

VERY LARGE ᢒᢌ Shaw tells a story of the bright family of children, now grown to university age, taking their old nurse to see *Hamlet,* and then coming out discussing the madness of Ophelia and the irresolution of Hamlet, finally turning to their old nurse to ask what she thought of the play. "I thought it was very sad," she answered. My abiding impression of America is an old nurse's one: I thought it was very large.   A. T. P., 1951

LITTLE THINGS ᢒᢌ Little things, like the clever landscaping on the Merritt Parkway, Howard Johnson's restaurants, the first banana-split we had ever had—or seen. Little things, because it was during those early, joyful weeks that our eyes and ears were alert and receptive to the trivial, thrilling detail of the New World: a grey squirrel at a bus stop, the siren of a fire-engine, a robin, a Negro child buying a Coke at the drugstore.

R. Q., 1952

NEW YORK: THE DEEP END ह‌ He who would make a "behind the scenes" approach to the United States would be well advised to put ashore at some quiet port in Maine or New Hampshire, travel south by slow stages, and finally, after a month or two in the backwoods, attempt New York City. But to arrive in the city direct is to go in at the deep end. It is to experience the physical shock of "Americanism," to be dazzled, fascinated, bewildered, and even revolted by the sheer glare and weight of it all. It is to stand in Times Square at night and say, with the ludicrous authority of the newly arrived, "Here is America, vulgar, materialistic, unashamed!" Toothpicks in the mouths of over-nourished diners, the prodigious weight and bulk of the daily newspaper, the half-smoked cigarettes in the gutters, the sidewalks mottled with rejected chewing gum—all this is an offence and a shock to the nervous system! It is the first shock of discovering how the other half of the world lives and of being reminded at every turn and at every sight in the streets that you are no longer standing outside but are actually, for the first time, inside.   D. G., 1951

NEW YORK: FRENZY ह‌ At first, I found New York a confusing and almost frantic city, and I missed the open spaces and haphazard arrangement of London. But New York is without question the most dynamic place in which I have lived, a city which endows its people with endless energy and enthusiasm. Perhaps this is the result of the fusion of so many races, nations, and cultures in so small a space. At times New York was too overwhelming and for a little while I had to escape from its frantic turmoil. But always, when I was away from New York I felt anew its great attractions, and going back has always been a happy and welcome event. New Yorkers are a strangely assorted crowd, voluble, temperamental, and in the grip of a highly competitive system. A subway rush-hour crowd is a fearsome mob, but I am told that during the Christmas blizzard a new, or more probably a latent, spirit came over the New Yorkers. "They took things calmly, and behaved like decent human beings. It's as if they can behave sensibly when something bigger than they are comes along; but when they are up against only another New Yorker whom they suspect of trying to get ahead of them, or in some way to outsmart them, then they are like inhabitants of the jungle." This tallies well with my own impressions: individually or at home, New Yorkers are some of the world's most lovable and hospitable folk.   R. B., 1947

NEW YORK: TIMES SQUARE ৯ It seemed to me that my quiet life of study and research had been monastic indeed as I gazed up at the gargantuan nudity of the figures on Mr. Bond's remarkable sign in Times Square.   R. Q., 1952

EARLY STARTING ৯ It was after leaving Washington, D.C., that we began to take real account of the weather, and plan our drive accordingly. We would get up bright and early, be hitched up and on the road by 6:45 or 7 A.M., and stop for breakfast about 9, sixty or seventy miles on. Then on again till noon, when we'd hole up for a spell, unless our destination were uncommon close. We have on occasion arrived at the end of the day's quota of miles by 1 or 2 P.M., but usually we made it by 4 or thereabouts. This gave us a long evening for a stroll, delightfully unencumbered by clothes or responsibilities, in the cool, balmy end of the day, listening to the bull-frogs and insect life, winding up with an ice-cold Coke from the gas-station. This was the time of year, and of day, when front porches are put to their proper use, as I remember stoeps being used in South Africa, for sitting out on in the dark, sipping something and just yarning. We have no front porches to speak of in Britain, and when it gets dark we draw curtains to keep it out. . . .

Even yet I bear the mark of these early morning drives southwards. As I was seated on the left-hand side of the car, and as the sun invariably shone and invariably from our left, my left arm was burned a far deeper shade of tan than my right arm.

A. D., 1952

NEW ORLEANS ॐ New Orleans fascinated us. Its character was distinctly un-American: although Chicago and New York have greater foreign and even non-English-speaking populations, their dominant culture is unmistakably Anglo-Saxon and Protestant; New Orleans, even to the indifferent observer, is palpably different. We thrilled to the sound of small boys fighting in French and were scandalized by the advertising along Rue Bourbon. Basin Street and Canal Street were to us legendary places out of the history of jazz—not to be thought of as actual *streets;* yet the reality did not bring disillusionment. We had a meal to soft candlelit music in the Court of the Two Sisters; and in the ancient cathedral we felt the continental Catholic atmosphere— an air of being unthinkingly Catholic that Ireland and Spain have; which is accompanied, however, by a distressingly evident lack of devotion, especially in the unashamed commercialization of the cathedral guides' concession. A. D., 1952

THE NEW SOUTH ॐ As we approached Gadsden and Birmingham, Alabama, the night sky flickered with the flares from the steel works. Everything was thriving and we wondered whether the poverty of the South was a myth. The farming people on the bus said they got all they wanted from the land, and one gathered that the amount of available cash needed in the country is much less than in the towns. C. H. W. M., 1948

THE SOUTHERN DREAM ॐ The radio spoke of a blizzard in New York, raging at Christmas time, but in Louisiana we had a mild sun and poinsettias, and winter was unimaginable. A clear yet curious scene, brown, dusty, and also brilliant, far different from anything I had known—though it was a dozen novels of the South

made actual. We drove along wide and quiet roads. Sometimes
there were bayous, that made one think of snakes, coiled in the
opaque water; sometimes thick acres of sugarcane, Negroes load-
ing bundles of cane into railroad cars.

As we went north the clock went backward. In St. Francisville
there was a churchyard, full of live oaks weirdly hung with grey
Spanish moss—that strange fungus that droops from Southern
trees. Tears, strands of hair gone grey, old trappings in a dusty
ballroom, tattered and forgotten flags—Spanish moss suggests all
these things. How could the South have won the War Between
the States, with Spanish moss for décor?

Under the trees, two Negroes dug a grave, laughing as they
turned up the brown earth. A bank of flowers near them shone
richly in a patch of sunlight. Two white children squatted against
the flowers, watching the men at work, whispering and grinning
at one another. The moss moved gently in the faintest of breezes.
Suddenly the scene was unreal—a vivid flash from a dream, every
colour heightened as in dreams. . . .

The unreality persisted as we went on towards Natchez. There
was no traffic on the straight road, and no one to be seen except
two white boys with a shotgun, a Negro family walking at the
road edge in single file, an old Negro with a wheelbarrow. We
found a Sibelius symphony on the car radio and, drunk with
music, drove in a delirium of speed, devouring distance in a
vacuum out of time. Only on the outskirts of Natchez did we
slow down, except for one small town where there were the
usual Negro hovels outside all other dwellings. Outside one,
like another flash from dreams, stood a Christmas-tree, twice as
high as the wretched cabin and all decked with tinsel and orna-
ments. There was great gallantry in such disproportionate
splendour.

In Natchez the first people we saw were a group of girls on
a lawn, all in long ante-bellum dresses, their hair in side-ringlets.
Dream again—though we found that they had only gathered

there for a publicity photo. Natchez is high on a bluff above the Mississippi, a town of a few thousand people living on the past. Before the Civil War it was a fashionable centre. There are nearly eighty ante-bellum mansions in or near it; some grand, some very beautiful. Most of them are occupied by rich southerners; the few intruders seem to have been long enough in occupation to be accepted. M. F. C., 1949

THE SOUTH: A SAD MYSTERY ‽ The flatness of the Midwest under leaden, wintry skies was something of an anticlimax, which was however amply compensated at Easter by the exciting experience of leaving Ann Arbor with snow still falling on bare trees, to drive southwards through Ohio and Kentucky (where the trees were a green haze of buds) into Tennessee where spring awaited us in its full glory of dogwood, purple Judas blossom, and leaves of the most delicate green. Not even the engineering wonders of the Norris Dam, not even seeing seven States from Look-Out Mountain could exceed the wonder of having gone to meet one spring—and then returning to await another one, equally beautiful, a short time later in Michigan. We cast a puzzled eye on decrepit shacks studding the hillside, with occasionally a tin bath hanging on one of the outside walls; we watched slim, jean-clad men leisurely following their mule-teams, ploughing ill-kept, barren-looking fields, and wondered at these and other signs of a low standard of life and habit in a land otherwise energetically prosperous. The South remained something of a sad mystery to us, as I suspect it is to the majority of Americans too. But we remember the courtesy of its farewell—"Hurry along back"— the glory of the Smokies and of Washington in her magnificent bridal dress of cherry blossom, and these things are neither sad nor mysterious. R. Q., 1952

THE STORY OF BIG LICK, TENNESSEE ‽ Big Lick (population about 300) lies in wooded country, part of the great T.V.A.

domain, some fourteen miles south of the small market town of Crossville. For two years the Rev. Eugene Smathers, a young Presbyterian minister, had preached on a four-point circuit in Cumberland County with little apparent result. Then in 1934, at the height of the depression's distress, he turned his back on the opportunity of preaching in a "high-steepled city church" and decided instead to move into Big Lick, one of his four points, and devote his life to the service of this little community of some fifty desperately poor and discouraged families. He is still there, although time has made him rather famous (he has an honorary doctorate from a great university). In true Church of Scotland tradition he has combined hard work on the land with a deep and thorough learning. When I first met him and Mrs. Smathers, he was busily at work as a mason on an extension to his house.

It is difficult now that things have changed so greatly to visualize just how poor and backward such communities were. The average cash income per family was little more than £12 and for six months of the year the roads were almost impassable. When anyone got sick, they waited till it was too late to call a doctor. Even so, it took a quarter of a year's income to pay for one call and people sometimes had to mortgage a cow to get a doctor to drive those fourteen miles. The majority of homes were without books and the average house had a value in the region of £100. There was every problem of poverty and undernourishment, both in body and mind.

Mr. Smathers first tried to tackle the problem of low incomes by bringing in expert agriculturalists. These made no impression and he almost decided that the people had no wish to solve their problems. Later it occurred to him that his agricultural experts had been trying to tell his people how to solve their problems instead of getting them to help themselves and discover their own problems. So he organized two study clubs meeting weekly. One group met in a home on one side of the parish and the second group on the opposite side, both on the same Wednesday night.

There were three notable results in the first year: the men got a new sense of their own ability to do something about their poverty; they learned to mix their own fertilizers and thus save money; and thirdly they formed a cooperative of twelve members, called the "Farmers' Association," to purchase farm machinery. Further developments followed in quick succession and the next problem was to get more farm land. The answer was a "homestead plan" in which Mr. Smathers and three laymen acted as trustees. It enabled a total of twenty-two families to buy their own holdings in the first three years.

During the spring of 1943, the community was selected as a demonstration area in soil conservation with the State College and the Tennessee Valley Authority sponsoring and directing the project. Then the community decided that the school house would no longer do as a "preaching place" and that they must have a church. Every home was canvassed and asked how many days of labour each would give and how many loads of stone. In seven months, by "workings," they completed their new church. One man gave as many as 114 days. The pastor acted as foreman and worked 140 days. Another problem was the health situation and there is now a health centre constructed in much the same way.

There are no signs now of the early struggles and poverty. Big Lick has become part of the hard-working prosperity so typical of the present-day rural America. Its resources have been greatly increased and diversified. New industries in the area, such as the great atomic plant at Oak Ridge some 40 miles away, together with the automobile, have brought alternative sources of income. Rural electrification (thanks to the T.V.A.) and the coming of the deep-freeze had made possible the easy and profitable marketing of such crops as strawberries and vegetables. Before this, Big Lick had been too far off the beaten track, too lacking in skills, altogether too unsure of itself, to compete in production of this kind. Of course problems still exist, but Mr.

Smathers and his parishioners remain firmly convinced that it is "better to light a candle than to curse the darkness."

F. P. C., 1953

THE BIBLE BELT ࢦ The Director was an alert, spare man, and looked like a Welshman. Actually he was of German origin, and left his farm to become Director. As befitted a director in the Bible Belt, there was a Bible on his desk for all to see. I soon found that it stood not only for no drinking, no smoking, no immorality, but, above all, for no damnyankees.

C. H. W. M., 1948

OHIO: LAPUTA ࢦ I visited Ohio and saw my first shoulder-roofed barn and some late fields of corn, which to a European visitor so confuse the sense of scale, seeming at first glance like fields of waist-high wheat instead of—as befits a big country—head-high maize.

A. P. S., 1952

CROSSING THE CENTRAL VALLEY ࢦ We drove out through Kentucky, Indiana, Illinois, Missouri, and Kansas, and returned through South Dakota, Minnesota, Wisconsin, Michigan, and Ohio: two thin and hurried threads drawn across half a continent. The best that can be done in such circumstances is to quote from the diary I kept, so as to have at any rate a succession of small scenes before one's eye:

"Inscription on a library cornerstone in Huntington, West Virginia:

THAT OUR SONS AND DAUGHTERS

MAY BE

AS CORNER STONES

POLISHED AFTER THE SIMILITUDE

OF A PALACE

Wondered why the inscription struck me; why you would only find such sentiments expressed thus in America. Not merely because the wording is unfelicitous—plenty of monuments in Britain offend worse—but because of its belief in education, its aspiration, its desire for 'polish'—i.e. for a successful worldliness on a par with New York. . . ."

"*Vincennes, Indiana:* Rather like Huntington, only smaller and hotter; how hot—88° at 9:30 P.M.—is indicated with a certain macabre emphasis by a floodlit thermometer outside the Gardner Mortuary. Worth more attention than Huntington, however, for its past—a French settlement that has given it its name and a handsome Catholic cathedral (three white figures illuminated in blue niches on a brick west front—Della Robbia effect): then Fort Sackville, captured from the British in the Revolutionary War by George Rogers Clark, after a remarkable march through the wilds. Easy to feel the frontier loneliness of Fort Sackville when you stand at night on the river bank and watch the Wabash sliding by, broad, black and treacly, in a silence mitigated only by the shrill, perpetual noise of crickets. Then a train howls in the dark and the spell is broken. In the town, stultifying smallness. Three movies showing bad films. Many neon signs. Shops straining to be go-ahead. Youths and girls on street-corners, in the thinnest of clothes; Elks lounging on their clubhouse porch, cigars and stale anecdotes, and neither fear nor excitement offered by tomorrow. . . ."

"*Salina, Kansas:* Another town of 20,000 or so, like so many others east of the Rockies and north of the Mason-Dixon line. You know that you are approaching them because the hoardings thicken at the roadside—billboards advertising hotels, motels, garages, churches. Perhaps a drive-in theatre (an open-air cinema which you watch from your car: the film is projected on to a high white wall that looks something like a war-memorial). Then, on the town outskirts, diners, gas-stations, motels, and always signs listing the clubs—Rotarians, Lions, Elks, Kiwanis, etc. Then streets of white frame houses, each with a porch, detached but not without hedges or railings. Streets called after trees or famous Americans. Then Main Street: a ragged skyline, rows of cars parked on either side, shops, more garages, bars, drugstores, movies, 'hamburger heavens.' A Greek-temple bank. The whole brilliantly lit at night by neon signs. Elsewhere in the town, a high school, a large white honor board listing the names of those who served in World War II (these boards furnish an excellent quick guide to the composition of the town, from the proportion of German or Scandinavian or Scotch-Irish names), and churches —Lutheran, Wesleyan Methodist, Methodist Episcopal, Congregational, Christian Science, Baptist, Seventh-Day Adventist, Jehovah's Witnesses. . . .

"As you go west, the towns become newer, more garish. You find fewer brick or stone buildings, and the graveyards become emptier and more marbly. There are no villages in the European sense, only disappointed townships. Rosebud, Kiro, and McGurk proved to be nothing more than a gas-station and a few houses clustered by the road edge as if by accident. The cities, though, are vigorous enough. St. Louis, on the west bank of the Mississippi, has much to commend it—an open-air municipal opera with a large number of free seats, a big park, a first-rate art gallery, and bold schemes for a civic centre on cleared ground by the river. Kansas City has a remarkable country club district, with eleven shopping centres, each in its own architectural style, without recourse to the monotonous if convenient checkerboard plan of so many American towns, beautifully laid out, with many trees, fountains and good (imported) statuary—so many trees in fact that, from the top of the Liberty Memorial, you can see little of the district except a green carpet of tree-tops, with here and there a red-tiled roof. The rest of Kansas City, from the same monument, is brash new buildings that struck dismay into me, so much did they resemble the crude, highly tinted postcards that make any town look soulless, and which for some reason, Americans seem to accept as representations of their homeland. . . ."

"On the road, eastern Kansas: Dull day, threatening rain; the sky enormous, mottled and lumpy, sagging, like the underneath of an endless mattress. The road and railway run together, with a spawn of telegraph poles and wires. The railway came first; the towns are more interested in it today. Only the garages cater for the road, the other buildings turn their back and consult the railway. Not that there are many buildings; oil-tanks, a grain elevator, a few sheds and houses.

"The view, ahead and behind, to left and right, is of minutely undulating wheatland, sparsely sprinkled with farms. Each farm is: a house, a wind-pump, half a dozen trees, a silo or two, a barn. In the vast fields, an occasional tractor, with a sunshade to protect the driver.

"The road: straight because it has no reason to curve, inviting speed, inducing sleep. Squashed turtles. A sign pointing off along a farm lane to a 'Beauty Shoppe,' though no sign of the shoppe. White grain silos stand up ahead over the Kansas skyline, seen miles away, like windmills and churches in the Netherlands. Tall, graceful, severe, they have the air of monuments—and are the region's only monuments, commemorating the annual abundance of grain. . . ."

And then, coming eastward, some weeks later:

"La Crosse, Wisconsin: Just into Wisconsin by the width of the Mississippi, which advances along the valley in great breadth, even so far north, a smooth and completely adult river. Drove 450 miles today, across part of South Dakota and all of southern Minnesota. The way was through rolling country, without hills until the last few miles before the Mississippi. Treeless until Mitchell, South Dakota, then increasingly verdurous. Rich farmland, green and golden hued, with corn and cut wheat, with now and then a welcome small lake to break the comfortable monotony. The sun shone all day.

"We've decisively left the West—those dusty, sprawling settlements that look like war-time camps, impermanent and undomesticated. Have come to more secure, more sedate places, with stone buildings going back as much as 80 years (a few months ago I should have written that as a joke, but in America one comes very quickly to accept a different time-chart from the European; 80 years is a long time here). These towns are less alien than the ones in Wyoming or Dakota, and yet make less appeal to one. They are the places where you need to wear a tie to eat in a restaurant, and where they cease to offer you a second cup of coffee. Two lines of demarcation—the Continental Divide along the Rockies, and then further east, the line of the Second Free Cup. We have crossed it. . . ."

"*Madison, Wisconsin:* When we left La Crosse for Madison, we were in good humour. Wisconsin breathed an atmosphere of briskness and liberalism—neat farms, admirable roads. Saw high corn; threshers blowing out chaff; handsome herds of cows. . . . Stopped for petrol a few miles north of Spring Green. The garage man was lively and loquacious: 'Well, I'll spend the morning cleaning up my station; this afternoon I'll tidy up the office and varnish my desk; then I'll go fishing; then this evening I'll get good and drunk.' He was doing well in his garage, he told us; certainly he seemed to have no doubts as to what constituted the Good Life. . . ."

I could write out many more extracts from my travel notes, but they would not add very much. This was the Central Valley, into which you could tuck England several times over. The tourist, appalled by the distances that confront him, covers it with his foot flat down, with glazed eyes and stifled yawn. He is heading for home or a holiday and the flat states bore him. They bored us, except for pleasant interludes, for we too were longing for the fabulous West. I remember now size, quantity, straight roads, trains racing the traffic, things growing, desperately optimistic little towns and genuinely optimistic big ones. It is the heartland but to me only in a geopolitical sense, however large and important an area it is. The bigness defeats the traveller;

only the inhabitant can feel at home as Willa Cather did. To him, far horizons are exhilarating; to the traveller they are only more miles to cover before night comes and the motels are full.

M. F. C., 1949

MINNESOTANS ☙ Some Minnesotans are such enthusiasts for their lake scenery that they are prepared to come out of their lovely heated houses in the middle of below-zero winter, and sit for hours in a little shelter on the ice, just thinking and drinking it all in. They are supposed to be fishing through a hole in the ice, but though we passed many of these colonies we never saw any fish! A. D., 1952

SALT LAKE CITY ☙ Salt Lake City itself we first saw by twilight. I suppose I had expected some signs of rigour in the headquarters of a people who take neither tobacco, alcohol, nor even tea. But at first glimpse it was like any other city in America: a rectangular pattern of wide streets, a multitude of hotels, motels, restaurants, fashionable shops, neon signs, movie-theatres, many cars, well-dressed pedestrians. . . . This was evidently a city that had prospered.

Next day's sightseeing confirmed the initial impressions of modernity and well-being, but added special Mormon overtones. With many other tourists—Salt Lake City is an enormous draw; present-day Mormons benefit from Gentile travellers just as did the Saints of a hundred years back, sitting on a transcontinental route—we made our way to the ten-acre Temple Square, within which are enclosed the principal Mormon buildings—The Tabernacle, the Temple, the Seagull Monument, the Assembly Hall, the first house in Utah (a crude log cabin, now incongruously sheltered beneath a classical pergola). The tourist traffic was highly organized; everywhere bunches of visitors were listening to guides, their heads swivelling obediently to and fro to take in each successive object. We found ourselves committed to the care of a genial and informative gentleman quite unlike the typical guide. He was, he told us, a lawyer. Every member of the church offered some service—his own voluntary and unpaid work was to explain Temple Square to visitors. And so we went into the vast hump-backed Tabernacle, listened in silence while a pin was dropped at its far end, to demonstrate the miraculous acoustics; stood around the Seagull Monument, while our lawyer friend told us of the plague of locusts that had threatened Utah until the Lord providentially sent seagulls to eat them up—since when the seagull has been a sort of sacred bird in Utah; eyed the log cabin; admired the flower beds and lawns, among which water-sprinklers turned; and gathered outside the Temple, which no Gentile may enter. Here was Mormonism symbolized, in a great grey cathedral, a plain, ugly, singular construction, like no other church I had ever seen. The guide told us something of it; how the Saints had determined to build a church that should last forever; how they designed it themselves; how it had been begun in sandstone until, after ten years' work had been done, Brigham Young found granite, when the sandstone walls were torn down to make way for the more enduring stone; how the glass for the 3,600 windows had had to be brought across the plains, pane by pane; how it had been forty years in the making.

M. F. C., 1949

CALIFORNIAN PARADISE ₰ Many English people go to California. It seems miraculous that they ever return. This is no land of lotus eaters, admittedly, but, apart from a few frenetic areas, it is like a foretaste of Paradise. Less studied than Italy, that experienced *femme fatale*, California is open, naive, delightful. Some day we shall come there to live. J. F. M., 1951

CROCK OF GOLD ₰ It was inevitable that the Joad family, "Okies" in Steinbeck's *Grapes of Wrath*, should head for California when their dust-bowl farm blew away. For California is the last repository of the American Dream, the ultimate in westering, the still-fabulous land to which the uprooted turn. A visit to California is one of the prime ambitions of millions of Americans; it is a shining place to them, an Avalon. There the sun shines, oranges hang upon the trees; there one's boisterous cousin went some fifteen years ago—he's got a good business, house with a lovely garden, and two fine children. . . . A haven for the old as well; Uncle Bill retired there and hasn't had rheumatism since. . . .

California, in short, is a state of mind, one of the new and buoyant places. Americans, when they are free to move, go now in search of what "California" implies—the sun, beaches, fruit-trees, work and playground combined. It is a state of mind that comprehends Florida as well as some of California's neighbour States—Nevada, Texas, New Mexico, and Arizona—which may not have beaches but where with civilization you can build swimming pools and air-conditioned homes and create green lawns, all the more delightful for the contrast offered by the encircling desert. All these States show the most spectacular recent rises in population, Florida 29 per cent between 1930 and 1940, California 22 per cent. The statistics of success could be multiplied without difficulty. One automobile firm, for example, states that there are more motorcars in California than in England, France, and Italy combined. . . .

This is the dream; the reality is of course more complex. There are several Californias. You can divide it into a southern section with Los Angeles for capital, a central whose chief city is San Francisco, and a northern, much more thinly populated, the "Redwood Empire" of giant trees, and vineyards. Or on a west-east division, there is the thin strip, crowded between the ocean and the coastal range of hills; beyond them the great valley of the centre (Sacramento, San Joaquin); and further inland still, the parched Sierras. Beaches and orchards, then dry hills, then flat food-producing valleys, and finally the ghost towns—Virginia

City, Fiddletown, Chinese Camp, Bodie, Havilah—collapsing quietly in queer corners among the mountains. Where could you find more diversity than in California, where, as they will tell you with understandable pride, you can swim in the warm waters of the Pacific in the morning and then get in your car and go skiing in the afternoon?

It is in fact a place for the young and for the old; for those who crave the sunshine, and who if they want snow must go and look for it in the mountains. A place also for the wanderer; where everybody is a newcomer, nobody can be an outsider; where nobody is a native, everybody is one. That, at any rate, is the theory.

Reactions to California tend to be violent. I never made up my mind whether I liked or loathed it. The worst side could be all summed up around Los Angeles, "the nineteen suburbs in search of a metropolis," of which Frank Lloyd Wright is supposed to have said that "if you tip the whole country sideways, Los Angeles is the place where everything loose will fall." Its architecture is a polyglot assembly; it has weird religious sects and small-animal hospitals; to the south sprout oil-derricks in monstrous jungles. It has the Forest Lawn cemetery, "with its Wee Kirk o' the Heather, Little Church of Flowers, and the remarkable stained glass window of 'The Last Supper' (phone for reservations)." It has Hollywood. Within a relatively small area are crowded enough freakish phenomena to keep a satirical novelist busy for a lifetime. No wonder that Aldous Huxley and Evelyn Waugh have taken their toll.

But there are other sides to California—qualities that kept Aldous Huxley living there after he had scourged it. There, and in the other States where there is no winter, it is possible to live in the sun, to eat prodigally and cheaply, even to drink reasonable California wine without paying much for it. There, you can live on the fringe of a desert, and yet live comfortably, achieving the impossible mixture of luxury and simplicity, with a car in the garage and drinks in the ice-box. In California you can find magnificent libraries, excellent universities, first-rate art collections. And there is San Francisco, as different from Los Angeles as Hamlet's father from his uncle. San Francisco perches on hills between the Bay and the Pacific Ocean, with two lovely bridges, remarkably good restaurants, and an agreeable air of bygone vice that links it with New Orleans in my memory. The mist severs the tops of the hills; the cable-cars master impossible gradients; from the Top of the Mark ladies peer down upon the world and—with a comfortable shudder—ask their escorts, "Which island is Alcatraz?" "Here," a bus-driver in San Francisco told us, "geraniums are weeds. You just let them have some water and they keep on coming up all the year round." If you admire such profusion in life, it is difficult not to like California.

M. F. C., 1949

Los Angeles: Heaven and Hell Ꮛᎈ Oddly enough, the single scene that I think the most beautiful of all that I saw in the United States I saw near Los Angeles, of all places. We had just dropped down into the Los Angeles–San Bernadino area from the desert (and nothing in California is more remarkable than the speed of the transition from dry brown desert to damp green coast) and one fellow got out at his home, literally in the midst of the orange groves, near Pomona. I looked around me, and there, near-by and all around, the golden oranges hung on the green, thickly leaved trees, while beyond, almost over our heads, the mountains rose up into the pale blue sky, themselves sprinkled lightly with snow and, with the sun on them, an exquisite, almost electric blue. That was very lovely, and such a contrast to the dreary waste of Los Angeles, into which—a little like Dante—I shortly plunged.   A. J. Y., 1948

Los Angeles: Possible and Likely Ꮛᎈ I was told in New York that Los Angeles was a wilderness of palm-lined boulevards, a

Pacific extension of Iowa, a mushroom growth in the desert, yet
I found it none of these things. It is true that Los Angeles typi-
fied for me much that seemed specifically American—rapid
growth, newness for its own sake, the culture of coffee-bar and
drugstore, an element of callousness that accompanies unchecked
competition—but these impressions are mellowed by the golden
Californian sunshine. Perhaps my most vivid memory is of getting
up each day in Beverly Hills to be greeted by a morning like the
most perfect sunlit spring day in England, and of feeling, amongst
healthy, happy people who crowded the streets, that anything
was possible, and even likely.   J. H. R., 1947

GOD, GOLD, AND THE PUEBLOS ?❧ Most of the elements that I
thought "typical" of the Southwest could be pointed out in Santa
Fe or Gallup. In Santa Fe the adobe style reigns supreme. It
was deposed for a while, last century, when Archbishop Lamy
built his cathedral in stone on European lines; and it has chal-
lenges from a sort of modified Spanish style—as in the Scottish
Rite Cathedral, which by one of those bizarre shifts in American
culture, is almost an exact reproduction of the Court of Lions in
the Alhambra, Granada. Otherwise, adobe is favourite—for the
post office, even for the electric laundry. Gallup, as a newer town,
has adopted modern variants. In both towns the railroad plays
a great part; the El Navajo Hotel in Gallup is built beside the
tracks, and the tall trains of the AT and SF (Atcheson, Topeka
and Santa Fe) dominate the town when they go through, with
such a splendid mourning of hooters and clanging of bells. Both
are tourist towns, with a rash of curio shops peddling cowboy
outfits, Navajo jewellery, rugs, and baskets, ashtrays and gaudy
Kachina dolls. Both are cattle towns, especially Gallup; like the
rest of the West they seem to demand cowboy films, a fact which
surprised us at first, until we reflected that a film about New York,
or Henry V, would convey very little to them. In both is to be
seen the medley of elements of the Southwest. Take, for example,

a Navajo bracelet, made of silver and turquoise. The Spanish taught the Indians to work silver; the Spanish are gone; the Navajo sell their craftsmanship to the American. Or take an Indian cowboy, riding near Gallup on his pony. The Spanish brought the horse to America; the Americans brought the cattle-herds; the cowboy, who speaks perhaps his own tongue, and perhaps Spanish, and wears his hair in a Navajo bun beneath a store Stetson, thus mingles three cultures. For the Indians, a coloured blanket; for the Spanish a church; for the Americans the railroad. Altar and locomotive were dynamic; the blanket, on the other hand, suggests repose, infolding of the spirit. The Indian could not withstand them, but he can win small victories. He can stay away from church; he can bump out to his pueblo in an automobile, while the whites buy his blankets and his portrait, painted by the simple-lifers of Taos and Santa Fe. The victory lies in the fact that while the tourists may admire him, he despises the tourists.   M. F. C., 1949

DESERT TOWNS ☙ The deserts of Arizona are fearful places, and it was fascinating to see the improvement wrought by man in bringing civilization to bear on them. I am thinking of the desert town on the main highway, consisting as it does of a regular linear arrangement: first a mile of hoardings, then a row of motels, a couple of used car lots and a set of gas-stations, followed by a bunch of cafes, a set of gas-stations, a couple more used car lots, another row of motels, and finally the backs of another mile of hoardings on the other side of the road. While not admiring these features individually, I was glad enough to profit by most of them when passing through, though I could never quite understand why each community was so fully equipped for the sale and ex-change of so many automobiles. It will be interesting to follow through the years the history of such towns which have no life of their own, but prey (not, as a rule, unfairly) on the passing wayfarer.   D. V. O., 1951

GARDEN OF THE GODS ﻬ We stayed in Colorado Springs and next day motored up Pikes Peak and then visited the Garden of the Gods. Where else but in the United States would one find a motor road, solely for pleasure, running to the top of a 14,109-foot-high mountain? And where else would one be able to purchase hot dogs, ice cream and picture postcards at the top?

G. A. S., 1949

TEXAS: SIZE ﻬ In Texas we decided to visit San Antonio instead of taking the shorter route across the Panhandle. The visit was remarkable not only for the beauty of the town and the interest of the Mexican influences and problems, but also for the very vivid experiences of remoteness. We seemed to be four hundred miles from anywhere; we could visualize Texas, but it was difficult to think in terms of the United States, and special concentration was required to remember Europe. We find that a large-scale gas-station map of southern Texas is a useful source of revelation in the matter of space to people in England, but the actual feeling of remoteness, and the on-the-ground register of distances and their implications can only be fully realized by covering the distances. We certainly find that our sympathy with the isolationism of, for example, the drugstore man in Big Springs is now something more than a detached intellectual understanding.

R. V. O., 1952

TEXANS PLEASE SKIP ﻬ Texas is the biggest state, the biggest producer of corn, cotton, pigs, cattle, oil, and liars, in the United States.

A. D., 1952

THE NATIONAL PARKS SERVICE ﻬ The American people can be grateful to the men whose efforts have preserved these areas for the nation and who have built up such a fine service to take care of them. The National Parks Service impressed me very much indeed. The officials whom I met appeared to be very soundly trained and to be extremely conscientious and keen in carrying out their duties. I was surprised at the apparent high standard of education of National Park men whom I met at isolated museums and offices of various parks.

I was interested in the efforts of the Service to educate the people on all aspects of natural history. The publications which are given or sold cheaply to the public are excellent, and I was greatly impressed by the many very fine museums which the National Parks Service maintains. All these things make it so very easy for an American who is interested in the geology, plants, or animals of his country to obtain, in a most pleasant manner, a very sound knowledge of these subjects. The lectures, the conducted tours, and the information service are all excellently designed for the same purpose. In short, the Service is doing a thoroughly scientific and important job in looking after the National Parks and in educating the people about their country. We have much to learn in Australia from these activities of the American people.

It costs a lot of money to administer the Service. Apart from the fees, the Parks produce no income other than rents from camps, hotels, and other establishments. There is no reason, however, why most Parks should not be self-supporting, in which case no admission fee would be necessary. They almost all have valuable forest resources and the bulk of these forests could be so managed under careful forestry practice that they would yield a large income without in any way impairing their beauty. Actually their scenic value could be thus increased.　　J. M. F., 1949

ONLY MAN IS VILE ఴ For one peaceful week on a deserted corner of String Lake we allowed the beauty of those spectacular snow-capped peaks, the crystal moraine lakes, the deserted woods which became alive if one sat still for minutes on end, and the chuckling mountain streams, to untie the complicated knots in our thinking and smooth our wrinkled brows. We were fortunate to meet some of the hardy folk who live in Jackson Hole throughout the year, and they shared their fine clean home with us. There was for me a surprising similarity in the thinking of these people to that of the deeply philosophical Scottish Highland crofters—a "sibness" we should call it. How surprising and profoundly disappointing to hear from them that in this most lovely valley where the evidence of God's handiwork is near to everyone, there is so much petty squabbling and jealousy among the residents that they have called it the "Valley of Dissension."

A. J. W., 1953

HOMUNCULUS ?❧ What a corrective to homocentricity it is! One talks glibly of five billion years, of the river flowing five thousand feet below, of the South Rim twenty-five miles' air-distance from the North Rim. But these are mere figures: one cannot grasp their meaning; one has no standards to measure by. These dimensions are completely outside of human scale. The city of Edinburgh is five miles air-distance from our home town, across the Firth of Forth; but it looks *much* farther away than does the North Rim from Yavupai. The same kind of thing may be said of El Capitan, the cliff of Yosemite which rises sheer from the valley to the preposterous height of three thousand feet. Now, Niagara manages to be just as impressive with much more man-size dimensions: Grand Canyon could have been just as visually grand if it had all been scaled down by two-thirds. Would we not have felt more at home with something we could understand? Does nature mock at the homunculus, or is it simply that the homunculus is irrelevant?

A. D., 1952

III. Academic Fields and the Universities

Universities

EDUCATION IN ITS ENVIRONMENT ᣸ Much has been written and no doubt will be written concerning the relative merits of our educational systems. The majority of critics appear to make the unpardonable mistake of taking one aspect of the system at random and comparing it, usually in an unfavourable light, with practices in their own country. The educational systems of all countries develop gradually in response to characteristics peculiar to the local environment. Whether the results achieved under the system within the particular environment are satisfactory or not becomes an argument of quite different character from that which springs from international comparisons.

It may be necessary to draw upon the experience of other countries in order to assess local merits, yet it is a disservice, in my opinion, to state categorically, "Your graduate system fails to produce the best results because it restricts individual freedom of study," without investigating the factors which moulded the system, a study which goes as far back as the kindergarten.

A. B. D., 1947

A GENERAL COMPARISON (1) ᣸ The entry standards at California (with 23,000 students) are appallingly low, and first-year students in America would have no hope of passing the university

88

entrance examination in Scotland. Thus it takes the American student, in my opinion, at least one year of graduate study to attain the level customary for a good honours student in Scotland. After that, the question becomes very difficult. In a sense, the American level never does come up to the British level, for California gives Ph.D.'s for work which would not be regarded as meriting this distinction in Great Britain. However, the very *style* of education is, on the graduate level, different from that at home. The American student must display a remarkable familiarity with the literature and techniques of his subject; it would be quite impossible for a student who had not recently been doing the "assigned reading" to answer many of the questions in a California preliminary exam—Lord Keynes himself, I am confident, could not have passed one without preparation. This compels the student to read widely, and a bright man cannot "get by" on rather scanty information. However, the system seems to me to have two disadvantages: firstly, it produces graduates who are well trained in following and repeating the ideas of other people, but not nearly so good at criticizing those ideas or producing any of their own—the type of mind which an Oxford professor described recently as being "able to fiddle cleverly with other peoples' ideas"; and secondly, it produces graduates who are experts in some branches of their subject but do not seem able, or do not seem to have been able to find the time (which may be more like it), to relate their specialized to their general knowledge. The British defect, I should say, is the opposite of all this —want of thoroughness, want of familiarity with the best work done elsewhere.

These criticisms, I think, are commonly made. What is less often remarked on is the reason for these differences between British and American education. The truth is, it seems to me, that the two systems are doing two essentially different things. The American university system is intended to provide a wide section of the population with a training which will enable them to do work of certain kinds—to be doctors, to be industrial engineers, to teach economics, to investigate social problems, and so on. In Great Britain, on the other hand, a university education is reserved for only one in every six hundred or so of the population, and is designed (as far as one can use the word about the vague, uncertain purposes characteristic of British institutions) to provide students with a training in how to think, and with some notion of the world about them and of how it is possible to visualize man's life in that world. I think that it would be less than honest not to add that I think the British (which is also the European) system to be superior; however, I also think that no comparison is fair which does not take into account the wide availability of a university education in America.

A. J. Y., 1948

A GENERAL COMPARISON (2) ₴❧ One cannot live long in the United States without realizing that education is a serious business. There appears to be, at least to British eyes, an undue urgency in completing the process of education whilst at the university. This sense of urgency arises out of two facts which are peculiar to American life. First, once one gets away from the eastern seaboard, towns may be very small and the distances between townships and indeed between homesteads may be very large. The opportunities for further education that exist in Britain through extension courses and the existence of good libraries within easy reach of most people, do not occur in the United States. Furthermore, the very rapid pace of American life leaves little room for further education after leaving the university. These two facts combine in my view to explain, at any rate in part, this sense of urgency on the part of the American undergraduate.

The standard attained by undergraduates in the American universities is frequently criticized in Britain. This criticism is often unjust inasmuch as it assumes that university education in both countries is attempting to attain the same objects. Owing to the low standard attained by the American high schools it is not possible for the universities to aim at a high standard for the first degree, nor is it desirable in view of the very large numbers attempting to attain that standard. It is now becoming evident that an increase in the numbers of undergraduates produces an over-all lowering of standards. At the graduate level the standards are more comparable with those attained in a British university. The graduate student spends approximately a year and a half attending formal lectures, after which he takes his Master's examination, which corresponds to an honours examination of a British university. The remaining year and a half of the three years' course are spent in research work. This is a rather shorter period than that normally spent in Britain, but nevertheless the quality of the graduates at the Ph.D. level is very nearly the same. It will be evident that I am not over-critical of the American system of university education, since I have attempted to understand its special problems. It is easy to come back from the United States an Evelyn Waugh (see *The Loved One*), much harder to become a Kenneth Harris (see *Travelling Tongues*); but I prefer the latter's viewpoint and believe it to be correct.   D. O. J., 1949

GOWNS WILL BE WORN ào There had been a considerable domestic crisis the previous term when it was decided that at dinner in Procter Hall, starting in September 1953, "Gowns will be worn." In Cambridge such an order might have read, "Gentlemen are requested to wear gowns," but the implicit note of authority would have been just as clearly understood. One was surprised on this occasion at how violently the American students reacted to what seemed a reasonable disciplinary action—gowns had been worn for many years until war-time restrictions had made the practice undesirable. "Discipline," it seemed to me, was the key word. A large meeting was convened which took the form of a one-sided debate in which the cleverest speakers could scarcely hide the fact that no one wanted gowns. An Irish friend of mine who made the mild suggestion that the graduate students were young whippersnappers and ought to do what they were told, was in grave danger for days.

In my limited experience, from the age when an American child is able to understand what it means to switch off a television set, or even to go to bed, he is slightly different from his British cousin. Perhaps there is a hereditary quality; indeed it is true that parents inherit a way of training their children. Whatever the explanation, it does not come easily to the average American to give unthinking, unquestioning obedience to a doubtful authority (and which authority is not doubtful?). We have been told in this country that "your policemen are simply wonderful!" Though my attitude to the American policeman was near to wonder at times, I could never imagine an American citizen regarding one of his own police in the same exalted light. There is an almost complete lack of "party discipline" in American politics as we know it. "An American soldier," I was told one day at lunch by a serious graduate student, "is like this piece of spaghetti; you can lead him anywhere, but you can't push him at all." If any tradition is dear to the heart of an American it is that of freedom—nobler by far than the wearing of a piece of black-out material. And so we had interesting discussions at table about the comparative merits of wearing gowns. Never were discussions more clearly academic, for in September 1953, at dinner in Procter Hall, gowns were worn.   A. J. W., 1953

INTELLECTUAL FREEDOM ॐ It was impossible to mix long in American academic circles in 1952–1953 without recognizing that McCarthyism was the dominant topic of thought and conversation. I do not think my own views and discoveries in regard to this are sufficiently different from those of other British visitors to the U.S.A. with whom I discussed the matter for them to be worth setting forth in detail. I shall not therefore discuss whether or in what sense there has been a Communist plot in the U.S.A., nor shall I argue the legal or moral rights and wrongs of the relevant congressional investigations, loyalty oaths, trials, and dismissals. But it is quite evident that some of the intellectual freedoms to which we are accustomed in northwestern Europe tend to be restricted by certain current pressures in the U.S.A. Not that American intellectual work in the arts and sciences is any less painstaking because of this. The profundity of American historical scholarship and the crystalline rigour of American mathematical logic, for instance, have not suffered at all. Indeed, perhaps much of the intellectual energy which might otherwise go into unorthodox speculation or criticism tends to be devoted to research and development in fields where a man need have no fear that he is risking his livelihood.

Of course, university curricula are changed with much greater ease and frequency than in Britain, so that the pressure of academic conservatism is not felt so strongly. The reason for this is, I think, that departmental decisions are generally taken by a vote of all permanent members, young and old alike, not by the senior member alone. But in historical interpretation (as opposed to historical scholarship), in economic theory (as opposed to the construction of mathematical models or the collection of economic statistics), or in political philosophy (as opposed to the compilation of data about political institutions)—to mention three of the academic subjects most affected—restrictive pressures from outside the university are much stronger than in northwestern Europe. Constant protests by alumni, students, and students' parents, coupled with the general atmosphere of congressional investigations and newspaper publicity, are not without a cumulative effect on what is taught to this generation and hence what is passed on to the next. Harvard seems to be much less susceptible to these pressures than most other universities, but even while I was there a book was taken off a history department reading-list after protests that it was subversive.

I am inclined to think that the real struggle for intellectual freedom in the U.S.A. has yet to be fought. The eighteenth-century colonists fought successfully for political autonomy, but they had not the same need to battle an established church for their intellectual liberties. That battle had been already won for them by their ancestors in Britain or by their very act of emigration. If local American orthodoxies became oppressive, they could always migrate again, like the Mormons, to a town or territory where their particular brand of nonconformism met with less opposition. Hence Americans have always been brought up to take their intellectual freedom for granted, as a secure inheritance entailed on them by the Constitution, rather than as a trophy of battle requiring constant watch and ward for its retention. Outside university circles, indeed, few Americans seem seriously worried about the impact of McCarthyism on American intellectual life, or have any sympathy for the current predicament of university teachers, whereas in northwestern Europe a similar attack on academic independence would raise up, I think, a much greater host of allies for the universities. Moreover, with the disappearance of the frontier and the rapid integration of American life under modern conditions the old refuges for the unorthodox have disappeared. I do not see, therefore, how American intellectuals can hope to secure their freedom (though there may be occasional lulls in the activity of their persecutors) until their compatriots are less obsessed by the fear of economic slumps and Russian aggression, which may not be for a century or more. Meanwhile, I think it the duty of all European visitors to the U.S.A. to bear witness—even at the risk of seeming self-righteous —to the present plight of intellectual life there. For liberty sometimes slides too slowly from a country for most of its natives to notice its disappearance.

Perhaps I should add, lest I seem one-sided on the issue of McCarthyism versus the universities, that an American professor can hardly expect perfect tolerance from his political opponents, when they come to power, unless he has kept his own party feelings out of lectures to his students. I was continually struck

during the presidential election campaign in 1952 by the openness
with which many professors of sociology, economics, or political
science surrendered the secrecy of their own ballot in efforts to
influence their students'. Nor did I ever hear it suggested by any
American professor, young or old, that there was anything un-
professional in this conduct. After all, if the academic profession
has special rights, it must also have special duties, and I do not
think American professors will ever be secure in the former until
they exhibit a higher degree of political objectivity within the
teacher-pupil relationship. Academic freedom is always inclined
to vary inversely with professorial partiality.   L. J. C., 1953

YALE: HIGH SERIOUSNESS ⧉ One thing I missed at Yale, and was
very glad to miss: the tacit assumption that nowhere else in
the world really mattered very much, and that the activities of
most other universities were in some strange way vaguely amusing; a state of mind which certainly existed to some extent at
Oxford, and which I sometimes shared and sometimes found
oppressive. On the other hand—and this is perhaps the converse
of what has just been said—I missed at Yale a certain devil-may-
care say-what-you-please, a certain *flânerie*, which is a possible
virtue of academic societies and at least prevents them from
taking themselves too seriously. I would not say that American
universities take themselves too seriously, or that American undergraduates take themselves more seriously than their present-
day British equivalents; but I think that the points at which they
laugh at themselves are different. They take the use of their
time more seriously, it seems to me, and they certainly take their
football more seriously. They also take the relations between the
sexes more seriously, or at any rate the social activities in which
those relations express themselves. I should say too that the
University cynics of Yale take their cynicism more seriously than
they do in Britain. The net result of all this is an existence which
generates more emotional tension than we are accustomed to.
   While there may obviously be a bad side to all this, I was im-

pressed by the very widespread determination to plumb the depths—often the very sordid depths—of human experience, and I thought that, more than in Britain, people were ready to look elsewhere than in their own academic field for answers to their questions. I met a physicist who had taken a year off to study the relations of science and religion, and although this may look like a copy-book case it appeared to me typical of a much more general trend, at any rate at Yale. The interest in the writings of William Faulkner among people outside the English faculty, and the attempt to see the "spiritual significance" of what he is saying may have been just the contemporary Yale "cult"; but they seemed to me to be a good deal more than that. I had the strong if ill-defined impression that people were looking for something which would give them an insight into the problem of how to act and what to think in the contemporary world, and that their search was on a fairly deep spiritual level. I heard a certain amount of talk about "insecurity," and it was clear that this was not, or not only, a political quest, but something more far-reaching. I discussed this with a professor from an English university on our return voyage across the Atlantic. He too had heard a good deal about "insecurity," and as an agnostic said that he was baffled by it, and was not sure what this thing was of which people were afraid. I had an answer to this question, as a student of theology; but I am not certain that either of us fully understood what the issues were.

On the political level, and among the non-academic majority of the nation, it seemed to me that the immense and unwavering trust placed in the new President of the United States was a symptom of this feeling of insecurity: here was the man who would put an end to it. On the religious level, it is perhaps true that the great increase in the membership and the activities of the churches is partly due to this same feeling. But I would not want to over-stress it; the immensely exhilarating enthusiasm of the American people for their own land and way of life is still,

I am sure, the dominant impression received by the visitor from abroad.   R. A. S. B., 1953

PRINCETON: MERE MALES ﾞﾞ Princeton has no women. A minor matter, maybe, but one which seems to strangle much of Princeton's extra-curricular life. The undergraduates keep their week-ends for "dates," either going a hundred miles or more to the women's colleges or bringing their girls to Princeton. Since they have heavy assignments of reading and writing for their courses, and since they wish to keep their week-ends clear, they must work long hours on week-days. This leaves them no time—and little inducement, in the absence of women—to organize discussions, concerts, and other informal meetings during the week. The evening in Princeton is extraordinarily dead.   H. A. H., 1953

UNION THEOLOGICAL SEMINARY ﾞﾞ If the theological teaching of Union reflected its character as a bridge between the thought of the Old World and that of the New, the common life of the Seminary was an index to the vital traffic crossing and recrossing that bridge. One thinks of the many visits of Kagawa, Pastor Niemoller, Professor C. H. Dodd, and many others who have inspired the world-wide church and whose influence is confined neither to native country nor denomination alone. And when one thinks of the world-wide church, the live consciousness of which has been called the "great new fact of our time," one inevitably thinks of the students of Union Seminary. On my floor alone there were students from France, Portugal, Switzerland, Holland, Japan, India, Germany, and New Zealand. The remaining six floors were no less cosmopolitan. We live in an age accustomed to international gatherings but we tend to be sceptical of their real success. During my stay at Union Seminary I was constantly shocked into a delighted recognition of the reality of this "great new fact of our time" and of its meaning for the various branches of the church. In this respect, I can think of no higher tribute to pay to the Seminary and its American students, than simply to say that it is playing a vital and unique part in the life of the world church. To find a parallel perhaps one would have to go back to Geneva in the time of Calvin!

D. G., 1951

CHICAGO: TOWN AND GOWN ᏃᏰ The first puzzle is to know how the University of Chicago survives in that part of that city. Because a less likely place in which to find the humanities and sciences flourishing could not easily be imagined, at least not by anyone familiar with the external appearance and environment of, say, Oxford or Cambridge. It appears, however, that this first-rate university can thrive in its small island of respectable streets in the midst of one of the largest and poorest coloured neighbourhoods in the States. It has suffered slightly from this situation, perhaps, in one strange way. The city of Chicago is founded, and always has been founded, upon present needs and present conditions. It is in no sense a historically minded city, and the inhabitants are proud of what they are, not of what they have been. Only in such an atmosphere entirely free of historical associations could a community spring up from whose lips the name of Aristotle is rarely absent and whose delight is so markedly derived from things which are no longer of everyday use. In Boston, in Philadelphia, the real presence of history, in the material form of buildings, imparts an unavoidable historical sense which does not send its possessors flying to remote ages to escape the present. And so it may be that the University of Chicago exists as a reaction from the necessity otherwise of living in the present, the manifestly unsympathetic present. This may be irresponsible speculation, but the fact remains that we have a most unworldly university in a most worldly city.

The temptation, particularly if my theory is correct, would be to adopt an air of culture as an affectation designed to show as clearly as possible the independence of "Town and Gown," and in fact it is true that no pains are taken to conceal the interest taken in Higher Things. But this appearance is backed up by such a capacity for hard work and difficult thinking that no serious accusation of affectation can be sustained for a moment. The only adverse criticism of the arrangement is that the average student takes life too seriously. This visitor found a comparative absence, not only of sports—the history of this is too well known to be repeated—but also of all those clubs and societies which one would expect to spring up plentifully in an intelligent community. Among those few groups which have sprung up, it was good to see several forms of government in action, ranging from Perfect Despotism (the University Choir) through Benevolent Oligarchy (the Country Dancers) and Representative Government (the International House Committee) to Complete Democracy (an informal madrigal group). Of these examples, I need hardly say that the most democratic was outstandingly the least successful.   D. V. O., 1951

CHICAGO: THE LEGACY OF CHANCELLOR HUTCHINS ?∼ The University of Chicago insists on the importance of a general education for all students; it refuses to give degrees in subjects of a purely utilitarian variety; it has sapped away the foundation of the fraternity system; it has abolished football. According to Chancellor Hutchins, a university should be a place where people think and teach others to think. . . .

I was impressed by the thoroughness with which this work was done. For example, a seminar on Aristotle's *Politics* met two or three times a week during the term and went through the book word for word and sentence by sentence. No attempt was made to finish this book in one term if it involved skimping, and throughout emphasis was laid on what Aristotle meant rather than on where he can be found in error. This determined attempt to understand what an author is trying to say seemed to me a welcome change from the tendency in England, where the undergraduate in his first term's work on philosophy is often asked or expected to destroy or at any rate criticize the argument of a thinker who is presumably of some stature.

Secondly, I noticed that the average American student found difficulty in expressing his thoughts either viva voce or on paper. This I accounted, on inadequate evidence, to (a) not having had a classical education (by this I mean not having learnt Latin or Greek; and not having been taught by people who had learnt Latin or Greek), (b) lack of practice. I have no knowledge of American high school education, but I gather from conversations that relatively small emphasis was placed upon the construction of the English sentence and little practice was had in the writing of an essay. Certainly it is possible to get a B.A. degree in Chicago by answering yes and no questions which do not involve a single essay.

Thirdly, in spite of the importance attached to general education in Chicago, I found that most people reading philosophy as a post-graduate subject expected to teach it and were surprised when I said that I had no such intentions. . . .

Finally, in spite of the radical nature of Hutchins' reforms, the thesis still remains the basic educational test. The value of a thesis varies with different subjects. Certainly many students wasted two valuable years of education in writing about a topic which was a good subject for a thesis simply because its intrinsic significance was so small that no one had ever bothered about it.

M. B. C., 1948

M.I.T.: AN APPRAISAL ⁊᷑ There is no technology school or faculty in Great Britain which approaches M.I.T. in size, facilities, or numbers of eminent men engaged on teaching and research. The Institute accommodates some 5,000 students, of whom about 1,600 are engaged in graduate studies. About three million dollars are spent on independent research and twelve million on sponsored research each year. Although much greater in scale and in scope than the work which is carried out in British universities, the undergraduate teaching and the research training of graduate students are of the same nature and have the same objectives. By examining the organization of the graduate studies at M.I.T., I am sure many ideas can be obtained which would be of great value if adopted (perhaps in a slightly modified form) by British research schools.

The presence of a large number of men eminent in their own fields, all people who take a real interest in education and who are filled with enthusiasm for the work of the Institute, is by far the most important reason for its great success. It is difficult to say why such an outstanding group of people collected together in the one Institute. I would guess that in the first place it was the magnetism of a few senior professors which drew large numbers of young men of real ability to their laboratories. The appeal of working in such an intellectually stimulating atmosphere is probably still the main attraction. I feel sure that such an organization cannot be built up artificially by some agency allocating large sums of money with which to tempt a heterogeneous collection of people who they think will be suitable for various offices in a carefully planned hierarchy. It should not be inferred from this that the "working conditions" of the staff at M.I.T. are poor. In fact they are probably as good as, if not better than, any other place in the United States and on the junior levels are certainly better than in Great Britain. Compared with their British counterparts the staff have, in general, a lighter teaching load, more opportunity to supplement their income from consulting fees, more congenial surroundings and living accommodation, and more facilities to enable them to do good research work. Although it is frequently stated as official policy that advancement in British universities is determined primarily by the lecturer's contribution to the advancement of knowledge in his own subject, these are in practice usually rather empty sentiments, since every member of the staff receives an annual increment in his salary no matter what his activities have been during the year (it seems that a grave "moral misdemeanour" is the only thing that will halt this relentless rise to the "grade ceiling"). Usually the research merit factor can only be operated by the person concerned being fortunate enough to have the opportunity of offering his services to another university or research organization. I detected no evidence of the dead hand of the inflexible salary scale in the administration of M.I.T.

Instruction of graduates usually takes the form of prescribed lecture courses. In general these are of two types; those which provide an advanced knowledge in one aspect of a basic science (designed for students whose previous training primarily has been in, say, metallurgical subjects), and those which set out to provide a sound knowledge of a specialized subject (say, physical metallurgy to physicists and chemists who have elected to do research in metallurgy). It is sometimes supposed that these lecture courses are of a standard usually found in the Honours undergraduate courses at British universities. In many American universities this is probably true. At M.I.T. the standard is considerably higher, as evidenced by the fact that many British students with Honours degrees find that at M.I.T. they have to study very hard to produce a creditable performance in the examinations. In addition to the formal courses the M.I.T. graduate student is required to produce evidence of some proficiency in two foreign languages and to subject himself to an extensive written and oral examination of his general knowledge of metallurgical science. The languages do not usually present any difficulty since the standard is not very different from that usually expected in the British School Certificate examination. The general knowledge examinations are not easy. Extensive and intelligent reading of recent publications over a wide range of topics is expected.

The research achievements of the student are judged by the report of his supervisor, a published thesis, and an oral examination. I was in constant touch with the work of more than a dozen students at various stages of their thesis work and read a large number of theses which had been submitted in previous years. I have no doubt that the extent and the quality of the work expected and achieved is in every way comparable with that at any British university.   W. S. O., 1952

Science and Technology

SCIENCE HUMANIZED: CALTECH AND OXFORD ⧸ℰ⧹ The California Institute of Technology presents a somewhat unexpected aspect to anyone visiting it for the first time. Half hidden behind palms, olive groves, and orange trees, it resembles a restored Spanish mission more than the functional cubic blocks suggested by the title. On closer inspections such buildings are to be found, indeed they are unavoidable for certain purposes, and are not to be improved by moulding in a gothic shell or covering with a baroque façade, but their effect is mitigated by discreet tree planting and by the prominence given to other sections of the campus. Frequently, the intended use of a building imposes no particular restrictions on its design, and the architects, free from that dread of imitation which seems to inspire so much current building elsewhere, have achieved a style at once pleasant and in harmony with the surroundings.

Scientific and technical rigour is softened in other ways too. Caltech undergraduates are obliged to devote one quarter of their efforts to studies lying outside the scientific field. For this purpose a separate building is provided containing a general semi-recreational library, a collection of gramophone records and playing room, a hall for concert performances, a newsroom, and a number of classrooms and studies. Both M.I.T. and Caltech are well aware of the risks inherent in their entire concentration on scientific subjects. In an ordinary university, informal discussion and exchange of ideas between young people in the various faculties is sufficient to ensure that a basic general knowledge is carried over from the humanities to the science side; in an institution which is wholly devoted to scientific and technical subjects this calls for special planning. In fact, there is considerable scope for educational experiments (as, for instance, the M.I.T. course in History of Ideas) which could not easily be fitted into the conventional academic scheme of most universities. For the most part, though, the undergraduate at Caltech selects subjects in the usual range between economics and foreign literature and accumulates his units over the years. The system works fairly well. It fits easily enough into the comparatively unspecialized curriculum of the American undergraduate, and, if there is some resentment when a low grade in an "irrelevant" humanities course spoils an otherwise creditable average, this is the exception, and it is the type of mishap which must occasionally occur whenever a course of study is broad by more than one subject.

Almost inevitably, such extra courses involve additional work in a program which is already very full and which consists largely in the assimilation of facts. They probably occupy the time which an intelligent Oxford student could use more pleasantly and more profitably in discussion, in recreational reading, or in some undergraduate activity of a broadly cultural nature. Nevertheless, one might have difficulty in assembling a group of science students, at Oxford or elsewhere, who employed their leisure in such a creditable manner. The Caltech system of organized courses in the humanities, although perhaps mildly unfavourable in its effect on the exceptional student, does at least ensure some general degree of devotion to other than scientific studies amongst the many. This is all the more important since it is the majority, rather than the exceptionally gifted few, who ultimately fill those positions requiring ability in the handling of human relations as well as some technical skill. The majority of industrial scientists need, even more than the pure research worker, to possess that mental bric-à-brac of miscellaneous fact and myth, that passing knowledge of the *lieux communs* of history and of literature, which forms the cultural heritage of a nation, and which is the implicit basis, if not the actual currency, of a great deal of personal intercourse.

It is perhaps a natural consequence of a move from the Oxford to the Caltech environment that one's attention should be drawn to the problem of relations between the sciences and the humanities. Oxford is outstanding in its intolerance of scientists and their works, and it must be the only remaining institution of any size in which the humanists have such a clear numerical majority. At Caltech the roles are reversed, and if there is less of a ghetto for the minority, amounting to little more than a separate table in the lunch room, one may put it down to the contrast between British reserve and American gregariousness.

Oxford has, however, if somewhat disapprovingly, provided well for the science undergraduate, and partly through good organization, partly through freedom from organization, he gets as much from his three short-termed years as his American counterpart does from a more than adequately planned curriculum. The British student, building on two or three years of specialized work at school, finally reaches a position in which he could without embarrassment continue study at any university in the United States. This would, in fact, be the best fate which could befall him, and it is unfortunate that financial problems, and ignorance of such possibilities as do exist, prevent more prospective British graduates from enrolling in American graduate schools.

More usually a good student will stay on at the British university in which he passed his undergraduate years. For the first year he may remain spiritually on an undergraduate plane, but as the terms pass and former friends move on, he will find himself drifting into that chilly netherworld which is the only British equivalent to the American graduate school. It is a world which lacks the rich and varied social life of the undergraduate community, lacks its spurs and its incentives, and lies in lonely isolation beyond the organized social and academic framework.

In literary or historical studies this may turn out to be the best preparation for a life of fruitful scholarship. If formal education ends with the Final examinations, there is no risk that an original mind will be hampered by an arbitrary syllabus. But the problem in the sciences is a different one. A methodical understanding of the aims, the problems, and the position reached by modern experimental science is the necessary precondition for originality to manifest itself, and, unfortunately, most scientific subjects have now reached a degree of elaboration which puts this understanding some way beyond the reach of the newly fledged B.A. or B.Sc. This is frequently sensed by research students in their first few months, and they may make haphazard and intermittent attempts to organize their further education on a private scale; but, without the examinational stimulus, assisted by competent direction, such plans are liable to drift through postponement to dereliction. The good intention ultimately reduces itself to attendance at one or two lectures arranged for post-graduate students, aided by the desultory perusal of whatever texts lend themselves to a more or less casual approach. Of course, certain specific problems arising in the course of research do obtain much more thorough and detailed attention, but these are no substitute for a planned course of study and they do not necessarily lead to an appreciation of the fundamental problems confronting a certain branch of science.

It is very different from the general mood and the organization of an American graduate school. This is the beginning of a new and vital phase in the student's career rather than the continuation of an old and slightly outworn habit. The newly enrolled members come from a variety of different places on the North American continent, and are often exploring a new and entirely unfamiliar part of their country. They have the hope of turning from mere academic transcripts into persons of promise and consequence in their new environment. In the easy, gregarious surroundings of halls of residence, in classes, and in the campus canteen they begin the gradual transition from undergraduate life to the more independent status of responsible individual research workers. During the first year they may see very little of research, perhaps only ten or a dozen hours a week in the laboratory. (This is the time when the American graduate student overtakes his Oxford contemporary, who is slowly losing the academic advantage which he possessed at the time of the Final Honours examination.)

In the next year the American student will, if he survives a series of ruthlessly searching tests, make his gradual entry into laboratory research, and the number of his classes will dwindle until at the end of the third year he is attending no more than the usual weekly research seminars.

I should qualify this by saying that my own first-hand knowledge of an American graduate school may not be in any way typical, since I have only seen the system working in scientific subjects (for which it seems to be particularly well adapted), and I was observing an unusual and outstanding example. In particular I do not know whether the close and friendly relations between the members of the Faculty and of the Graduate School, which so impressed me at the beginning of my stay at Caltech, are the general rule in most universities or whether they are exceptional. But I should guess that the social vitality and intellectual alertness in the Caltech graduate school might be paralleled in many similar establishments, and that these qualities are inherent in the nature of the institution itself.

W. B. M., 1953

SCIENCE IS KING I came to the University of California from a very small university where the hall-mark of a really able and well-educated individual is the ability to read Latin and Greek; those who cannot read Latin and Greek may, it is felt, be able people, but are not quite of the top rank. At Cal (as Matthew Arnold would have said) "this is not quite so." Cal is a decidedly 20th-century university: there, it is the mathematicians who are the intellectual élite; after them, the physicists; then the chemists; then—a long way behind—the botanists and biologists; and last of all, the intellectual riff-raff, those whose doubtful abilities are devoted to such subjects as literature, economics, psychology, sociology, history, and so forth. Physics at Cal is pretty well the official religion and the big red-roofed temple up the hill is there to prove it. Thus at Cal I entered an intellectual world entirely new to me, challenging all my previous ideas about the importance of literary subjects and of the literary approach to any subject. At one point I was even driven to studying algebra, on my own, furtively, in the engineering library.

A. J. Y., 1948

RESEARCH PROBLEMS (1)୫ I feel that one thing is having a bad effect in many ways on United States scientists: the pressing need to publish results quickly to keep their names to the forefront because competition is keen for the better positions and often the number of publications counts rather than the quality.

The emphasis then is on the publication of small pieces of research without waiting for a year or two until more data are accumulated and a better picture of the problem in question is obtained. Often the little pieces of research have to be written so guardedly that they don't convey the impression of sound work and many hypotheses built from a poor scaffold are put forward which have no real bearing on the facts. A general tightening up by editorial staffs on the various journals would help to check this trend. Often a research worker, pressed for publications, may take the route in his work which will lead to a partial result quickly, whereas with extra time to think it over the apparently less fruitful approach would in the end lead to greater success. This emphasis on research publications has also the effect of making directors of research institutes tend to employ postdoctoral or trained staff rather than spend time in training a post-graduate student who will require attention during his period of training and will not be in a position to produce results for some time.

Against all this it may be said that competition between rival laboratories among such a large group of workers is so keen that a worker must be thorough to avoid serious criticism by his fellows.   J. G., 1950

RESEARCH PROBLEMS (2) ৯৯ Another of the sources of misdirected research is the fact that in some schools only two years' work or less is required for the Ph.D. degree, a further year or so being taken up with various kinds of course work. The supply of simple problems capable of solution in two years is very limited, and consequently the research student is unlikely to step outside a fairly narrow range of problems for fear of embarking upon a project which will lead to nothing in about eighteen months. It is almost axiomatic that research intended for a thesis will be designed to produce the greatest possible impression rather than to further the state of science, but this evil is much aggravated by the shortness of time available.

Perhaps the greatest factor contributing to American success in this field, or for that matter in any field, is the invincible combination of energy and enthusiasm with which so many workers attack their problems. This virtue in the research student enables him to defeat the limitations of his short term of work as far as these can be defeated at all, and in the senior staff sets a tone and pace to the whole laboratory, including the assistant staff, which conquers all material difficulties on the spot.

A second notable feature is the use of new materials and techniques for handling them. The enterprise of manufacturers has not only brought a wide variety of plastics, ceramics, and alloys into being, but has placed them at the disposal of the research worker in quantity and in all those forms in which they are most wanted. Machinists and scientists alike have been quick to take advantage of this situation, and have not been afraid to do the necessary pioneer work.

The division between experimental and theoretical physicists is becoming harder and harder to bridge because of the more recent mathematical techniques available to the latter. As a result, the theoretician is permitted to hide behind his smoke screen of new functions and operators, and, when he occasionally sticks out his hand waving a new prediction, there is a rush to investigate experimentally without asking him where he found it and what he proposes to do about it when it comes back marked "Yes" or "No." Science might progress in this way, though to the detriment of the education of all concerned, were it not for the fact that the prediction so often comes back from the experimentalist marked "Zqp" or "Xg." "Ah," says the theoretician, "you have *not* disproved my theory. I shall write a letter to the *Philosophical Magazine* (or to the *Physical Review*) about this." And so he does, dammit, so he does!   D. V. O., 1951

THE SAD FATE OF THE SCIENTIFIC PH.D. ﹠ In so far as a generalization is possible the British Ph.D. tends to regard an industrial career as a lower calling than one of pure research, and to find the nature of industrial work irksome after the freedom of his graduate period. He is more suited to independence of research and to academic work. It is not surprising, as opportunities of such work are relatively few, to find discontent among "those who failed to avoid industry." America would appear to equip many more chemists far better for a happy and useful career in industry, the main field of employment of the Ph.D.

From the faculty viewpoint, the state of affairs is different. The English academic is likely to be more favourably placed than the American. The latter, has, of course, to make a relatively greater financial sacrifice than the Briton. A Ph.D. entering industry now commences at $6,000 per annum; an instructor receives $4,000, and a full professor less than $7,000. But a more important reason may well be the less favourable structure of the American university from the viewpoint of its teachers. The American teacher perhaps feels himself less as being the university, and more the hired employee of the university, with his promotion (genuinely important if real hardship is not to result) in the hands of persons judging him mainly by the quantity of his publications. Results of the quest for promotion are the high mobility of teachers from university to university, and the tendency of professors other than the most senior to plan research primarily in the light of the probability of publication of the outcome. Cases exemplifying these principles which I have seen include an assistant professor of rare ability as a teacher and counselor having to enter industrial employment because his rather low rate of publication denied him promotion; a full professor who in order to reach this position had been a faculty member of four universities in six years; a theoretical chemist who four years after producing his first paper, one of considerable consequence to the subject of catalysis, has now begun producing at a great rate, but matter almost wholly useless.

B. M. W. T., 1951

PRINCETON MATHEMATICS ᙇᙄ If one takes into account the combined influence of the powerful Princeton University Mathematics Department and of the Institute for Advanced Study, Princeton must be one of the first few centres of mathematical research in the world. The average Cambridge undergraduate is convinced that he is being introduced to the most abstract and the most up-to-date mathematics, but he would be surprised to hear the reaction of the average Princeton graduate student to the Mathematical Tripos. It is fair to add that many of the best Princeton mathematicians admit that they cannot do the Tripos questions; but it does not worry them. The approach in the American universities (and here I am only talking of the advanced work) is more abstract and brings the student into contact with the outstanding research problems at a much earlier stage. In Cambridge a student has to look for his research supervisor in some obscure garret in a college tower, whereas in Princeton everyone chats to several professors at tea in Fine Hall. However, there is a certain ruthlessness behind this informality at Princeton, and a student who is not progressing with his Ph.D. research is apt to become more quickly distressed than his equally neurotic Cambridge equivalent. There is a second good reason for his anxiety—the usual time taken to complete a Ph.D. thesis is rather less than two years after "Generals" and in Cambridge the minimum time is three years after "Part III." In other words the Cambridge man has almost twice as long as a research student and a late start is not so frightening. The Cambridge thesis is usually a good deal longer, and it was amusing to my American friends to see me struggle to send a large thesis back to Cambridge in June, travel three thousand miles for an oral in early September, and wait many anxious weeks till the degree was conferred (by proxy) in November. It seemed to be possible to burn the midnight oil in Princeton for a fortnight, to present the thesis to a professor on Saturday, have an oral on Monday afternoon, and celebrate the same evening. Princeton may not be sufficiently representative, but the American graduate students I have seen are harder working, better prepared, and more impressive mathematicians than my Cambridge friends.

In England there are only two universities whose mathematical status is comparable with that of Princeton—Cambridge and, to a lesser degree, Manchester. In the United States there must be a good dozen—Yale, Harvard, Chicago, Berkeley, to mention only a few. Mathematicians in Europe are only beginning to realize the tremendous strides the subject has made in America—it is time they did, for in this as in so many other fields of activity, she is becoming the leader of the world.

A. J. W., 1953

SPONSORED RESEARCH: A METALLURGIST'S ASSESSMENT ⅋ There is a general misconception in British university circles that the large sums of money that have been provided for research in the United States are spread thinly over a large number of universities and much of it is spent on work of a practical nature which is considered unsuitable for university study. . . .

Since most of the American work is financed through Government or industrial research projects, in most cases the work is organized on a large scale so that it is carried out by teams of people. These are usually directed by a senior member of the academic staff and contain from one to a dozen or more graduate students and, possibly, as many technicians.

There are very few examples of this type of organization in the British universities. All the significant British contributions to metallurgy in the last five years have been made by individual members of the academic staffs, perhaps working with the assistance of one or two graduate students and with almost no technical assistance. Thus, in general, the researches have been different in content and in experimental procedure. However, it should not be implied that individual initiative and opportunity are lacking in the American universities. All give a large measure of freedom to their staff to choose subjects of research. The money for small-scale experiments of the British type is readily available to those who require it. Many staff members participate in both types of research simultaneously. Furthermore, on the large-scale projects there is complete freedom to decide the theoretical and experimental attack on the problem being studied. As a result, much work of fundamental importance has come out of what at first sight might appear to be a very routine industrial type of problem. The universities are aware of the dangers concealed in sponsored research and are constantly vigilant to ensure that it does not result in their laboratories being employed to produce large quantities of empirical data which, while such data may be of immediate but transitory interest to the industry, are of little value in furthering our knowledge of the metallic state. They consider the empirical studies to be the province of the industrial laboratories. Thus, while both a university and an industrial laboratory may be studying what appears to be almost the same problem, their approach is quite different. The administrators of American universities consider that the large-scale project offers a number of advantages. It allows a large number of different experimental techniques to be used on the one problem so that very valuable experience is obtained by the graduate student in assessing, correlating, and using a variety of types of information. The over-all chance of success is greatly increased. Thus almost from the very beginning of his research period the student has the sense that he is participating in significant original work. He is working with a number of people who have a wide knowledge of the environment of the subject on which he is working, and thus he can obtain an accurate measure of the value of his results and a great deal of guidance and stimulation. This is especially important in the first two years of his work.

The large-scale research sponsored by the Government and industry in Great Britain is almost exclusively carried out either in Government laboratories or by the research associations. There is in America a certain amount of published work coming from Government laboratories, such as the Bureau of Standards, but there are no research associations of the British type. The available output from these sources is small compared with the British. It is of interest to compare the sponsored work in American universities with that in the British research associations. The latter organizations have also greatly increased in financial resources, equipment, and numbers of staff since the end of the war, but their contribution to the sciences of physical metallurgy has been very small compared with the American. Although these organizations, both in statements by their directors and in publications, make pious claims to have as one of their reasons for existence the pursuit of fundamental knowledge, they have in recent years been almost exclusively concerned with giving short-term service to industry. There are, of course, one or two notable exceptions to this statement.

In both countries the producers and users of metal have "research" laboratories which are solely organized and financed by individual industrial organizations. These primarily concern themselves with day-to-day problems, but some do carry out a limited amount of work of a fundamental nature. Of the metal-producing concerns there seems little to choose between the research work in the two countries, although it should be mentioned that the work of the United States Steel Research Laboratory at Kearney, New Jersey, is outstanding. Amongst the American metal-users there are several large organizations which have excellent laboratories in which fundamental work of a very high quality is carried out. The most outstanding of these are General Electric, Westinghouse, and Bell Telephone. Although several laboratories patterned on these models have been built in England, no work of comparable quantity or quality is being produced. . . .

To summarize, I think it is fair to say that within the subject of physical metallurgy many more important ideas and contributions to theoretical development and experimental techniques are now coming from the major American universities than from the British. I suggest that this is a reversal of the situation as it was fifteen or twenty years ago. However, in certain fields British work is still probably ahead; particularly those which are being developed by the use of electron theory and diffraction techniques.   W. S. O., 1952

Medicine

MEDICAL EDUCATION (1) ဠ During my stay I paid particular attention to certain aspects of medical education in the States. I went in the belief that, following his schooling, the student underwent an extremely liberal college course before entering his professional school, that the professional course was shorter than that pursued in England, and that the student then passed into his years of medical postgraduate training. The course would therefore appear well designed to discourage the early specialization so widely deplored in educational circles. But I found that these excellent intentions had been abandoned under the pressure of circumstances, especially the pressure of the hordes of students seeking to enter the medical schools. The competition is such that a student who has pursued a truly liberal education in his college course has no chance of entering a medical school because the places are filled by those who have already studied chemistry, physics, biology, mathematics, anatomy, and physiology with perhaps a bow towards liberality by a few semester hours of psychology, economics, or sociology. Thus the preclinical training differs little from that followed in England and indeed I think has the defect that these studies are not followed under the aegis of the medical school or integrated with them. In fact, valuable time is lost by repeating in the medical school work done in the college course, work now repeated with a specifically medical slant. Moreover, many students are unable to enter medical schools immediately after their college courses and have to wait one or more years—thus, to some extent, losing contact with medical subjects though many fill in their time profitably by assisting in research subjects. Further, an appreciable number cannot hope to enter a medical school which is connected with their college, but have to uproot themselves and move to a new centre.

There they plunge into four years of very intensive medical training based on short, intensive courses and pursued with such thoroughness that they have no time for anything else and would lose much of the benefit of a previous liberal education had they had one. This was perhaps the most striking thing I noticed while living at Duke, the tremendous concentration on work and the indifference to anything lying outside it. Though I was myself educated at a "Redbrick University" I can well remember the

amazing number of diverse interests of my fellow medical students, which I simply could not parallel at Duke, although I
tried to. (I do not think Duke was unique in this.) Nor do I think
the students benefited from this concentration, much of it imposed
by the severity of their intensive short courses. My own observation showed me that such courses became burdensome, and that
the student longed to get to the end of them, slam his books,
thank his gods that this course was over, and forget the bulk of
what he had learnt as he passed to a new course. Nor was he
ever required to remember and reproduce his knowledge in
detail, as there were neither departmental examinations nor any
final professional examinations to test his knowledge. In consequence it is impossible to compare or contrast the teaching
achievements of different medical schools.

It might be asked: with all these defects, why is American
medicine so good and its standards so high? I think the answer
lies in the quality and keenness of its students, the severity of the
competition in professional life and the excellence of the intern
and residency training years. For these I have the utmost admiration. My only doubt is that they are perhaps too severe and
impose too great a strain on the new M.D. Might not this be
eased by spreading the burden, by improving the courses in
earlier years and by more co-ordination of courses—as is being
done so well in Denver and in some other places? My general
criticism of what I saw of American education is that it is made
too easy for the schoolchildren and the college students and too
hard for the post-graduates. I think this is true of other professional fields, too, and I suspect that this has important repercussions. It was pointed out to me by a French scientist that the
increasing longevity of the American people as a whole is not
matched by an increasing longevity of its physicians and scientists, who are dying, to an extent that astonished me, relatively
young men, very often from disease of the heart. While no doubt
many factors play a part in this I cannot but suspect that the

immense strain of the post-graduate years must have some baleful effects, must take away some qualities of the tissues, must play its part in depriving the country of so many of its "elder statesmen" of medicine and science, who from their wisdom and experience might temper the prevailing pragmatism with some much-needed theory.

There are many features of medical education in the U.S.A. that are excellent, and some of these I shall hope to apply in the future. Nor are the defects I saw in American medical education unrealized there. On the contrary, I met widespread dissatisfaction; there is a critical atmosphere and a desire for change. The new curriculum at Denver and its excellent system of postgraduate education and the new approaches being thought out at the Western Reserve University at Cleveland are symptomatic of this.   J. N. P. D., 1950

MEDICAL EDUCATION (2) ਟ✎ In the traditional sense the old frontier days of the U.S.A. may have gone, but the pioneering spirit appears to have survived in the new frontiers of science. It engenders an attitude which colours the whole field of medicine in America. In the medical schools it accounts probably for some interesting teaching techniques which are not in such evidence in British schools. In the average British university the aim is to ensure that the medical student secures a thorough grasp of past medical achievements and proven knowledge. The teacher in America (I refer here to Harvard and Johns Hopkins chiefly) seemed to concentrate more on expounding what was *not* known about a subject. Such an approach presupposes that the student will on his own initiative consolidate his knowledge on more basic aspects—indeed, it is necessary for him to do so if he wishes to derive full advantage from the instruction offered. This supposition may not always be fulfilled and some American medical students may graduate with a less comprehensive background of knowledge than do their British counterparts. But

certainly it fosters an attitude of keen inquisitiveness and mini-
mizes the possibility of the student's completing his course with
a mind fogged by intellectual oedema and bereft of all enthusiasm, whatever its factual content.   J. D. R., 1951

NATIONAL HEALTH SERVICE ॐ Several times during our stay I
gave talks to doctors on the British National Health Service and
was always asked whether I thought such a health scheme was
necessary in the States. I said then and still maintain that more
good than harm would result from it for several reasons:

1. I am sure that there are people, especially Negroes, who
have to do without effective medical care because they cannot
afford it.

2. Doctors' bills are a cause for worry with the average man
in America.

3. The general practitioner is paid out of all proportion to
the effort involved. This is the greatest factor in the resistance to
socialized medicine as clearly demonstrated by the million-dollar
campaign against state medicine which the A.M.A. has just
completed.   D. R., 1951

PSYCHIATRY ॐ My tour covered most of the leading American
centres, and my impression was that they differed from advanced
British clinics in the following respects:

1. Their general concept of psychiatry as a basic science of
inter-personal relationships which permeates the whole field of
medicine, rather than existing as a narrow specialty.

2. The wide-spread enthusiastic acceptance of psychoanalytic
principles by both the profession and the public.

3. The highly sophisticated organization of the modern American psychiatric department with its close integration into the
working of a general hospital in many instances.

4. The emphasis on research techniques and usually the availability of trained men, plenty of money, and encouragement.

5. Enthusiasm about exploring borderlands between psychiatry and other disciplines; e.g., medicine, surgery, and obstetrics.

A. B. S., 1951

Political Science

POLITICAL SCIENCE IN AMERICA ૐ I do not think I am being purely autobiographical when I say that students of politics often find it hard to answer questions, however friendly in intention, on the nature, scope, or significance of their subject. An answer is complicated, to begin with, by the current division of the subject into political theory or philosophy (often regarded as a slightly illegitimate and not very important or fundamental aspect of moral philosophy) and political institutions (usually consisting of a legalistic, factual, and relatively unanalytic study of the governmental machinery of various countries). This, at least, tends to be the case in Britain, where the reigning confusion about the subject is reflected in the varying ways its teaching is organized in the universities: in a few cases there is a separate department of politics or political science; in others the theory side is taught in one or another of the philosophy departments, while the factual side, where it is taught at all, is likely to be taught within any one or all of the departments of history, economics, and law. And this is to leave out of account any mention of international relations, which may or may not be considered an aspect of politics.

In the United States most universities now have separate departments of politics, sometimes along with another department for international affairs. But within each department there will be a host of specialized courses or fields which frequently are taught in virtual isolation from one another. This too reflects a basic uncertainty as to what the study of politics, if there is any one study called "politics," is all about, other than that it is vaguely about "government." The one thing it does not seem to be concerned with is what the layman means by the term "politics." In a world beset by vital and unsolved political problems, almost the last people who seem to have anything important to contribute are teachers and students of politics in the universities. Hitherto, discussion of pressing political problems has tended to be the preserve of the propagandist or active politician rather than the scholar. I do not think this is too distorted a picture of the general and traditional state of political studies, and it is obviously somewhat unsatisfactory. However, some indications, at least, of how to improve on this situation are now being given in the U.S. . . .

Political science in the United States could be characterized in two ways: the approach was predominantly institutional, and tended towards increasing specialization. By the former characterization I mean that attention has been focussed mainly on formal, legal, relatively static and objective aspects of politics, upon constitutions, electoral processes, judicial interpretations, administrative structures, and so on. By the latter I mean that there has been a tendency to break down the subject into such separate fields as political parties, legislatures, public opinion, public administration, American government, and comparative government, all of which, in turn, are often further subdivided. This may be necessary as the body of factual knowledge increases, but too often the special fields become separate ones, trivia are over-emphasized, and the larger questions remain untouched, except briefly in concluding paragraphs, as lying beyond the scope of any one field. Now there are definite moves, here and there, away from the merely institutional in the direction of the more personal and dynamic, and away from specialization in the direction of what is being called the "interdisciplinary" approach.
. . .

At the moment, some of the devotees of this new interdisciplinary political science seem more or less content to accept the older focus of "government," if they consider the question at all. Partly this is because they are, at the moment, more interested in the methodological aspects of the subject than in the substantive ones. Such people are mainly interested in the question: "How would one set about dealing with a specific problem, if ever anyone were to set about dealing with it?" Only too often, the methodologists lay themselves open to the charge of erring in the direction of being interested in method virtually to the exclusion of an interest in content, or even of being devoid of any reference to it. For them, sociology and economics seem to be the main methodological models. One gains the impression from some of them that they have taken flight into methodology to avoid having to grapple with concrete problems and thus to avoid having to commit themselves on any issue of pressing public concern or upon which the board of trustees, or State Legislature, might be expected to have definite, and different, opinions.

Others have adopted this wider approach to political science simply because they have found it necessary in order to make headway with their studies of concrete problems. For them, the focus of political science is the study of power, and not only governmental power. According to this view, the central task of political science, and one distinguishing it from the other social sciences, is to examine the use of distribution of power among the various groups and individuals in society, and the ways in which this is conditioned by, and conditions, the nature of any given society. To me this is potentially the most significant and fruitful emphasis if political science is ever to become a systematic, coherent, and important body of knowledge. This conception of political science as a study of power, drawing upon the findings of the other social sciences was new to me, and is still comparatively novel (or even suspect) in this country. My introduction to it I count as one of the most important benefits of my stay at Princeton.

However, it is important to add that this whole interdisciplinary approach is still very much confined to a minority of American political scientists. To appreciate this fact one need only attend a meeting of any of the political science associations, from which one gains the impression that very little advance has been made in any direction in the past twenty years or so. On the other hand, the number is increasing, to judge by the reception given to Snyder and Wilson's *Roots of Political Behavior,* a book of readings designed as an introduction to political science. But, by and large, the number of people who accept the new approach, or who use it in their writings, is still very small. For this there are a number of fairly obvious reasons. To begin with there is a natural conservatism. This takes two forms: a plain reluctance to adopt a new idea; and a political conservatism which shies from some of the implications of, especially, the power emphasis. For one of the implications of the wider range of political inquiry must be that some of the myths and fables should be scrutinized and, in many cases, exposed. Further, a dynamic study of politics must examine the conditions for change and stability in a society, and the associated question of other possible forms of society or other ways of doing things may often smack of radicalism. This conservative attitude, is, of course, particularly rife under present conditions in America where, too often, the test applied to a teacher is not efficiency but loyalty to an orthodoxy defined by conservative groups.

Tentatively, I would suggest that the answer lies along these lines. In time, the social sciences will have to be recognized as a group of subjects separate from the liberal arts, just as are the natural sciences, so that a student at the university would devote the main part of his time to acquiring a basic knowledge of many of the social sciences, just as a budding chemist must study physics or biology, as well as chemistry, at some stage. Then, at later stages in his career, when specialization is necessary, the political scientist will choose some area within political science, if need be a fairly small area, but will study it in the light of what he knows or can learn about the relevant finds of other people and disciplines. Further, in working on any specific project, much more use than is now customary must be made of team work by a group of men with somewhat differing trainings. This may not solve all the difficulties, but it does seem to be the only answer. Finally, if the new approach can lead to more fruitful work in terms of more stimulating hypotheses and more inclusive generalizations, to that extent the problem can be rendered less acute than it is now amidst the welter of uncoordinated facts and theoretical conclusions.

If, in fact, political science should begin to add to one's knowledge of the political process and of the whys and wherefores of individual and group behaviour, a serious problem arises as to the use to which that knowledge is to be put. Obviously, the more that is known about human behaviour, the easier it is to manipulate men from the outside and for purposes which may or may not be generally considered as desirable. This is analogous to the questions asked themselves by many scientists working upon such things as atomic energy, who have begun to wonder whether or not they should concern themselves to a greater extent with the ends to which their discoveries will be devoted. In other words, shall political (and other social) scientists simply allow their skills and knowledge to be used by the highest bidder, as is already happening in that aspect of public-opinion studies known as public relations, or shall they insist that they be used for socially desired or desirable purposes? And, if the latter, who shall decide what are socially desirable purposes? This problem arises, in one form or another, with almost any branch of knowledge, but it seems to raise particularly acute moral problems when the issue at stake is the possible direct manipulation of human beings. At the very least, it suggests to me that some of the older forms of academic "impartiality" and "objectivity" might be out of place, if not positively dangerous, in the modern world.

G. C. M., 1950

The Humanities

THE HISTORY INDUSTRY ᙂ In general the English historian cannot help admiring the American approach to historical research. There is as well an element of repulsion when confronted with the endless bibliographies, card indexes, articles, and techniques which make many historical departments similar to factories. English scholars still prefer to work as individuals; the atmosphere of the cloistered college, the hermit at work among the folios remains to the Englishman the ideal for scholarly work, however much the reality has changed under the pressure of two world wars. The eccentric, the absent-minded professor is the image rooted in English tradition; whereas to the American, scholarly work almost approaches a business. This contrast can of course be overdone, and I for one was deeply impressed by American historical work. There is a wide-spread awareness that American history is in need of synthesis to combine the results of research with literary eloquence. The writings of Morison, Commager, and Nevins have shown the way.   W. A. B., 1952

CLASSICS IN AMERICA ᙂ There are many first-rate classical scholars in America, a fact not always recognized in England. Nevertheless, Classics is a dying subject there, more even than in England. Yet one of the most valuable results of my visit was the apprehension of the enthusiasm with which the specialists pursued their generally unappreciated studies, and of the firm conviction of their ultimate value. There is no cynicism about it; in England, classical scholars have not yet been forced back quite to the wall, and are consequently sometimes less certain. Not that the attitude in America belongs entirely to the ivory tower —on the contrary, a large effort is being made to adapt the teaching of Greek and Roman culture to the linguistic ignorance of the time, and scholars who are experts on the archaic inscriptions from the Acropolis or the events of 31 B.C. are making a successful job of lecturing in words of few syllables on Greek tragedy in translation. Sometimes the result is a comparatively worthless superficiality, which is the danger of all General Education, so-called; at Harvard I was particularly sceptical of the assumption, emanating in its worst form from Chicago, that an eighteen-year-old could, simply by reading selected works of Aeschylus, Virgil, Dante, Dostoievski, James Joyce, and the rest, attain to any real understanding of literature and culture. Illegitimate synthesis and exotic generalization are temptations which are not, I thought, always successfully resisted even by professors (and especially by instructors), at Harvard and elsewhere.   G. S. K., 1950

MEDIAEVAL STUDIES ᘐᕈ By any yard-stick, the most important work in mediaeval English literature is being done at Michigan with the compiling, editing, and publishing of the *Middle English Dictionary* which will be a basic tool in all mediaeval English studies, and the interpretation and appraisement of all mediaeval writings, whether in literature, historiography, law, science, or medicine. So far, no part of the *Dictionary* has actually appeared, but even in the fairly distant future when the last volume has been reviewed, Ann Arbor will still remain a place of pilgrimage for mediaevalists, since of course not more than a fraction of the two or three million quotations collected and filed will be published in the *Dictionary;* the rest of this mass of valuable archive material will remain available to researchers.   R. Q., 1952

RESEARCH PUBLICATIONS ᘐᕈ At every university and college I visited I was impressed by the quality and activity of the members of the faculty. Their energy and enthusiasm were infectious. Their ability to combine heavy teaching programs and continuous research, without loss to social and family life, was in many cases a revelation. One important incentive to the research was the need to publish in order to secure promotion or security of tenure. In a few cases this incentive is unfortunate: the faculty member publishes for the sake of publication and his teaching is adversely affected. For the majority, however, the incentive is stimulating and healthy and the teaching is improved by the infusion of the interest and findings of the research. Most of the men I met had written books and articles because they had something to say, and their research interest had been genuinely stimulated by the assurance that their research findings or their critical essays would be published. This assurance remarkably affects the conditions of study and writing. I was prompted by the American practice of writing and the assurance that there was an interested public and place for publication to prepare two articles which would in England have remained unformulated. In Britain there are only a few periodicals which are ready to accept literary critical articles, but in America an article of any worth is sure to come to rest in one of many possible periodicals. The scope of the university presses in the United States is considerably more ambitious than that of the presses in Britain, and a faculty member does not write his book in a publishing vacuum. There is, of course, the danger that men may easily publish unconsidered ideas and rush into print with the equivalent of the "bright notion" which comes as a suspiciously startling discovery late in the night's thinking and reading. Prolixity, as well as eccentricity, may be encouraged and long articles may grow into books, but the stimulus to study and the consequent beneficial effects on teaching are invaluable. Ideally, perhaps, literary criticism and research should not be affected by publication prospects, but human and even academic nature being what it is, I am sure that if British opportunities for publication were as numerous as those of America there would be a beneficial stimulus to both research and criticism.   R. V. O., 1952

WRITERS AS TEACHERS ᏖᏗ The American practice of including in the faculty of the English department a poet or novelist as teacher of creative writing is a practice which would be welcome in England. The student benefits appreciably by the attempt to write. Even if his writing is of little merit in itself, the attempt to write gives him an understanding and appreciation of literature which is direct in its nature; and the writing keeps alive in him the creative sense which is frequently lost in unrelieved British critical studies. The student is brought into touch with a creative writer and the practitioner's interest in literature. The writer is usually a man of more than usual alertness and life and his presence in the department brings an important contribution to its spirit; his influence is undefinable, but it extends well beyond the actual teaching of creative writing.   R. V. O., 1952

Law

PROFESSIONAL TRAINING IN THE UNIVERSITIES ?➤ The aims and objects of the American law school are very different from those of the faculties of law in the older English universities. We teach undergraduates and set out to give them an arts degree through the study of the law: this means inevitably that the approach is more academic, the area covered is smaller, and the more factual and unintellectual subjects are omitted and then taken at a later stage in the professional examinations. All students in England must spend time either in a barrister's chambers or in a solicitor's office as pupils before practising. American law schools have tackled the enormous task of teaching in school all the subjects that are needed for practice; they almost invariably take, as their students, college graduates. One cannot compare individual schools in England and America, as their aims and material are so different. And a comparison even between the two systems of teaching in England and America is unreal, as the English system is limited by the division of the profession into barristers and solicitors and by the custom, or in the case of solicitors, the requirement, of undergoing further practical training after graduation.

Without, therefore, going into details, I will offer one vital advantage of the American system. It ensures that every branch of legal study receives some academic attention; principles are discussed, and values of right and wrong maintained. We tend to treat academically the subjects selected for study in a university; practical subjects are learnt after leaving the university in order to pass the bar examination or the solicitor's final. There develops a difference between "academic" and "practical" law; the latter becomes too dependent upon form and precedent and too little dependent on principle. The result is that in many fields, particularly in subjects not taught at English universities, American law has solved many problems which the English courts have not even faced. My comments on the English system are referable particularly to the older universities. More practical courses are available at provincial universities and at the Inns of Court Law School. But these to a great extent rely on lectures for instruction, at the expense of discussion and argument which is the life-blood of legal teaching.   R. H. M., 1952

CRIMINAL LAW ॐ It very quickly became obvious to me that criminal law was not regarded as the most important of subjects in the Harvard Law School. One of the two lecturers in the subject described it as the Cinderella of legal studies, while the other found it necessary to make something of an apology for its inclusion in the first-year syllabus. Graduates of the Harvard Law School, he explained, would not expect to have much to do with the criminal law in their professional lives, but it was something that their friends would expect them, as lawyers, to know something about. They ought to be able to explain the technical details of the latest murder trial which was filling the headlines of newspapers. So, even though corporation and tax law were the important subjects which would enable them to earn their living, they should also know something of the criminal law.

This approach to the criminal law is not peculiar to Harvard, but seems to extend to most of the leading law schools of America.

It is an unfortunate fact that the defence of criminal cases is no longer regarded in the United States as entirely respectable.

The explanation seems to be largely an economic one. Persons accused of crime are usually poor, whereas those who engage in civil litigation are, as often as not, rich. The young lawyer who can obtain employment in a law firm or a corporation at a good salary is naturally not going to embark on a hazardous career at the criminal bar. Consequently the best of the nation's lawyers eschew criminal practice.

This is obviously not the whole explanation, for the same situation has not arisen in England, where criminal clients are at least equally poor and the lawyer is just as concerned with making money as his American brother. There are, in my opinion, two reasons for this: first, the division of the profession in England into solicitors and barristers; and second, the control exercised over the two branches of the profession by the Law Society and the Inns of Court respectively. The young barrister who wishes to practice cannot join a law firm at a salary: barristers are not permitted to form partnerships or companies. He must set out on his own, getting what briefs he can. The only cases which are likely to come his way so early in his career are criminal ones. Thus from the outset the young barrister becomes accustomed to defending—and prosecuting—criminal cases. The best young members of the common law bar compete for criminal briefs which not only bring in some badly needed money but also help the young man to make a reputation. The division of the profession, then, ensures that good men go into criminal practice. The strong professional tradition fostered and enforced by the Inns of Court ensures that their behaviour in practice will be of a high standard.

J. C. S., 1953

IV. American Life and Institutions

Politics

IDEALISM IN FOREIGN POLICY 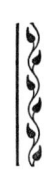 A tractor-driving farmer in South Dakota began by asking me when the British were going to stop taxing Canada and why they were so "soft" towards Communism, and ended an hour's discussion in his wheatfields by wanting me to write more to him about the achievements of Socialism in Britain and about the reasons why Mr. Churchill thought it might be worth talking with Mr. Malenkov. He began with all the prejudices bred by the capsule form of foreign news in mid-western newspapers and radio bulletins and by the public statements of his senators. But unlike them, he had no vested interest in hostility and he had a high degree of intelligence. He was willing and anxious to hear what I had to say, and in any event he took with a grain of salt what he heard both from his radio and from me.

Americans do not suffer from the disillusioned cynicism so common in Europe. One newspaper editor, after we had been discussing whether it would be tactically sound to withdraw Allied troops from Germany as part of a general agreement with Russia, broke in to ask, "But what is our moral duty? What ought we to do for the good of Germany as well as ourselves?" Another declined to discuss the coming negotiations with China in terms of practical expediency and would consider them only in ethical

131

terms. Good and bad, right and wrong are still very important to many Americans.   H. A. H., 1953

ISOLATIONISM ࿐ The immediate rewards of my tour of the country, the memory of staggering spectacle, frightening in the Bad Lands, ennobling at Mount Rushmore, thrilling in the Rocky Mountain National Park, have tended by their very immediacy to obscure the more subtle rewards of having glimpsed the life of cowboy, prospector, Mormon, and wheat farmer. But here is one thing I can now appreciate. If you are struggling with summer's searing heat or winter's pitiless fury on a South Dakota ranch where your dwelling is ten miles from the highway and fifty from a drugstore, the squabbles of tiny countries four thousand miles away in Europe will seem an irrelevant irritation to you. Isolationism has come to be used too much as a bad word, relating to Chicago press-lords and Ohio politicians, and instead of high-minded (and frequently unjust) indignation, some appreciation of the Midwest problems and some sympathy with the outlook of the men that face them would improve Europe's standing with these stout farmers and our relations with America in general.   R. Q., 1952

POLITICAL PARTIES ࿐ The basic design of political thinking seems fairly similar throughout the Western world. People support a given party for a wide variety of reasons: for hereditary reasons, in that they may uncritically accept the political views of their parents; for environmental reasons, in that they may happen to arrive at political maturity in, say, a period of depression, or again may climb (or fall) into a different layer of society from that which was hereditary with them, and may accordingly adapt their political views to those of their immediate communal associates; for psychological reasons, in that they may develop, whether from external or internal causes, some mental grudge against society so as to form a picture of themselves as underdogs or overlords; and most commonly of all, for economic or financial reasons—a perfectly unobjectionable ground if one regards politics realistically, but which it seems nevertheless conventional to treat as some sort of skeleton in the electoral closet, to be described, if at all, in the cosier phrase "enlightened self-interest."

Few voters vote as they do from any single one of these motives. Fewer still are capable or even desirous of analysing their own mixture of motives. So that it is fair to say that voting is on the whole an emotional process—not only, be it added, on the part of the elector, but also of the candidate in so far as his canvassing for votes influences the ultimate result.

It would, I think, be fair to add that advancing age (associated as it is in our pattern of society with a drive towards economic independence) tends to make the individual increasingly conservative. This, however, is not always to equate "conservative" with "right-wing," for those who (as I have instanced) happen to reach political maturity in a period when the pendulum swung leftward may crystallize in that attitude, so that we have the spectacle of, say, an Aneurin Bevan whose attitudes are still rooted in the class war of pre-1918 Britain; a New Dealer who still expects the banks to fail any minute; or a labour organizer in either country whose struggle for "better pay and conditions" has ceased to be motivated by crusading fervour and has become simply a justification of his own official existence.

Let me also say here, for the benefit of those who, like Walter Lippmann (the greatest American columnist?), deplore the mechanistic view of politics, that I am perfectly conscious that many voters make, or strive to make, an intellectual and unselfish approach to their political decisions. But (1) they are a minority and (2) in so far as their motives are then self-explanatory, they seem to me to require so much the less examination even by amateurish Dr. Watsons like myself.

Little purpose would be served by attempting to equate party labels in Britain and the United States. The British Liberal Party, still opinionatively strong though electorally negligible, has no precise equivalent, its attitudes being distributed (in much more powerful proportions) between Republicans and Democrats. The British Labour Party bears a certain correspondence to the left wing of the Democrats and shades off, as the American party did in 1948 into the Progressives, into a kind of no man's land between Socialism and Soviet Communism. But on the whole, the differences are greater than the similarities.

There is in Britain, for instance, no exact parallel with the conservative Democrat of the South. Although the leading labour affiliations declared for Stevenson, their association with the Democratic Party is much more remote than that between the British Labour Party and the Trades Union Congress. The Labour Party lacks the strong Catholic element in the Democratic Party. And the whole factor of racial minorities, so important in an American election, is largely (though not altogether in the major ports) absent in British politics.

But if the labels are forgotten, the individual voters appear to base their attitudes similarly enough. The farmer (traditionally conservative) will change his allegiance if his economic condition becomes serious enough and (if things then go sufficiently well with him) tend to return to his hereditary conservatism. The migrant to the city and to industry will be less conservative at the outset, but as and if he prospers and moves into the suburban commuting class will tend rightward. The immigrant to Eldorado will be leftish on arrival (if from Europe and not a refugee aristocrat) but may make an exaggerated swing towards the right if he feels it politic; as a result of McCarthyist pressure, for instance, or if he or his second generation "makes good" under free enterprise conditions. Those who are born rich (and free and white) will want to remain so and be inclined to vote Republican. In the South some who are born to none of these things will vote Republican because there the "have-not" party has traditionally been the Republican Party. Over this fluid sea of change wags the inexorable pendulum which dictates that when a party of the right is in power the left will build up support, and vice versa. Though American faith in the pendulum had been somewhat diminished by the Democrats' twenty years in office, its slow tick was still audible in the background.

A. P. S., 1952

PARTISAN ⁊⧫ Early in my stay I informed an acquaintance that I thought Roosevelt was one of the greatest men of the century, that Acheson would go down in history as the man who had forged the Western alliance against Communism, that I admired Truman and thought Stevenson the greatest statesman the West —including England—had produced. His reaction was to ask, "If you are so damned anti-American what are you doing here?"

E. R. R., 1953

THE CONVENTIONS ⁊⧫ As a political institution, the conventions seemed to me to rate a good deal higher than their general reputation allows. There is an element of tomfoolery—the Republicans seemed to have more money and energy to expend on helicopters and hotel-lobby excesses than the Democrats—and the convention-hall ovations are artificial, being controlled by the chairman and orchestra leader between them. But steam has to be blown off somehow, and everybody is excited.

What impressed me was that the delegates are really "little people" from all over the country, much fuller of responsibility than (as is commonly alleged) bourbon; and that a lot of hard and honest work is done behind the scenes in committee. It may be that, between the impact of television and the clear evidence (in the emergence of Eisenhower, Kefauver, and Stevenson) of popular antipathy to machine politics, the machine politicians held a looser rein than they had at previous conventions. But I had no earlier experience for purposes of comparison.

In any case, my impression was that in 1952, at least, the two best and most popular candidates for the presidency emerged at the end of two strenuous and dramatic weeks. (In fact, with the defeat of Republican neo-isolationism the election was in a sense already over.) The convention system seemed to me—in view of American geography and political traditions—good, and I should be sorry to see it hastily altered; some TV viewers, for instance, complained of the excessive length of speeches and too frequent polling of delegations. But the first is traditional, the second often a matter of political tactics, and both accordingly deserve more consideration than the arm-chair critic may be inclined to give them, forgetting that boredom is easily remedied by the turn of a switch on his receiving set.

As to the conventions' reputation for mass folly, it occurred to me that this may have been at least inflated by the press and radio. I saw in Alistair Cooke's company (though not in his material) enough of the reporter's desperate search for "picturesque" gossip—to lighten the heavier accounts of purely political manoeuvring—to suggest that the picture tends to be exaggerated simply because reportage is a highly competitive business and because, the public having come to expect eccentricities to be reported from the convention city, the supply must at all costs meet the demand.   A. P. S., 1952

THE QUICK ANSWER ಶಿ The quick answer shows up in ordinary conversation: it is "smart" to have a quick retort or a wisecrack on all occasions—and some of them are very good. It shows in offices, where everyone keeps his door open, which is practically a guarantee against creative thinking. It shows at its very worst in the sign-posted beauty spot, as in the beautiful Bellengrath Gardens near Mobile, Alabama, where, to save the time of the surface-skimming tourist, an unexpected view of a carpet of flowers across a charming little lake is labelled "Look."

In politics, too, the quick answer is paramount. As General

Marshall said good-humouredly in Korea in June 1951: "If we start an attack in the morning and don't have victory by the afternoon, in my country that's a stalemate." This easily leads to a lot of misunderstanding in international affairs, for that is a field in which quick answers are almost never attainable. The rest of the world is alarmed by the impatience of Americans. It fears that they, who in many ways are amazingly undeterred by the prospect of a third world war, will land everyone else in a global conflict at the drop of a hat. How often have we heard, especially in the Middle West, the exclamation, "Why don't we drop a few atom bombs on the Russians and get it over with?" The atom bomb is, of course, the ultimate expression of the quick answer and as such a horrifyingly attractive proposition to anyone who has a fallacious belief in the bomb's capacity to put a rapid end to the threat of Communism.

For this reason Americans will no doubt scare their friends for generations to come. If you are impatient you come quickly to a conclusion. If that conclusion is challenged, you resort to emotion. Emotion, however, is soon succeeded by reflection. The history of the MacArthur affair is an interesting case in point, not least (except for the actual method of dismissal) its skilful political handling by the Truman Administration and the speed with which the head of steam dissolved.

In all this, there seem to me to be two risks; first that under pressure of public opinion the critical decisions will be taken before the emotion evaporates, secondly that the policy resulting from the reflection will be cast in a form inadequate to appeal to the American love of the dramatic. In the main, however, American foreign policy in the last decade seems to have hit the nail squarely on the head a quite remarkable number of times and I believe that if the understanding between the United States and her allies can be strengthened by increasing contact at all levels there is little to fear.   A. A. P., 1951

BACKGROUND OF THE "WITCH-HUNT" ⧽~ The most striking and obvious contrast between British and American politics today is the injection into the latter of the anti-Red "witch-hunt," and, in fact, the American attitude towards Communism and Russia in general. The intensity of this American attitude seems to be quite out of proportion to the size and nature of the threat, so that it is not easy to understand what it is all about. Its very existence is sometimes surprising, when one remembers how extraordinarily interested in, and amenable to, criticism so many Americans seem to be. I was most impressed, for example, by the fact that I never made a critical comment that had not been made before me, frequently with much greater fervour, by some Americans.

The witch-hunt obviously is facilitated by the existence of the general pressure towards conformity in American society, and by the lack of an organized liberal movement. In the absence of a mass following, the liberal organizations can do little more than give aid to individual victims, even if often quite effectively. The labour movement has similarly offered no coherent or continuous opposition, partly because it shares the general antipathy towards Communism, partly because some union leaders have found it convenient to brand as Communist any opposition groups within their unions, and partly also because many labour leaders are still concerned with trying to appear "respectable"—just because they, in the past, have been called "un-American," now they try to prove that charge false by levying it against others. From labour's point of view, it is extremely doubtful whether it is pursuing the correct policy, given the known anti-labour views of the chief "hunters." The witch-hunt is also facilitated by the American political system, which allows so much power to such small, well-organized and well-financed groups as the China lobby, which has taken a leading role in the whole campaign. (It is worth noting, in passing, that the modern habit of referring to such groups as veto-groups is frequently misleading, in so far

as the name suggests that the power they wield is only negative.)
In this context, the upshot of the system is to permit a group of
politicians to follow a policy, with important results, which the
leaders of neither major party would be willing, officially, to
endorse, but which they are unable to prevent even if they wished
to. That under some circumstances this might be considered as
an advantage is irrelevant to the point at issue, for the effect
has been simply to allow plenty of scope to a vicious and cor-
rupting campaign.

But these factors, in themselves, do little to explain the grip
which the witch-hunters have obtained on American life. Given
the campaign's origin with a small group, the China lobby, and
the "hundred-per-centers"; given Truman's decision not to com-
bat it directly but rather, through the Administration's loyalty
program set up under Executive Order 9835 of 1947, to try to
head it off by meeting it half-way; given the factors already mentioned; and given, also, the legitimate concern over the defence
against espionage, there would seem to be at least three other
major influences which must be noted if one is even to begin
to understand how it has reached its present proportions.

First, of course, is the Cold War (including its hottest part,
Korea). So long as it lasts and the United States continues to
regard Russia and China as the Enemy, with whose leaders and
ideology there can be no real settlement, for just so long, probably, will the witch-hunt last too—a grim prospect. For, so it is
argued, there is no point fighting to contain Communism abroad
while allowing the slightest trace of it to contaminate the homeland—even though, one might add, the result is often just to copy
the methods of the enemy. Force and mobilization, it is said, can
be met only with force and mobilization—and evil with evil?
From this point of view the drive for "loyalty" and against
"subversives" can probably be best understood as a reflection of
American fears and expectations of war at the same time as it
is a psychological preparation for war, inducing that similarity

of outlook and conviction of righteousness that seem indispensable to belligerence. But no one, to my knowledge, thinks that America is in danger of being invaded and attacked by Liberals and Socialists. The main reason why the witch-hunt has been extended to cover many of them too consists not simply in a failure to distinguish them from Communists; rather, it is a direct outcome of the second major influence, to be discussed forthwith.

. . .

If, as has frequently been maintained, the New Deal constituted a revolution, with its different conception about the relative roles of labour, government, and business, then the witch-hunt can be seen as a manifestation of the corresponding counter-revolution. In other words, the present preoccupation with orthodoxy, subversive ideas, and defending the American way of life, combined with the attempt to identify "Americanism" with "free enterprise," is a product of the unease, the pangs of insecurity, felt by the defenders of the existing economic system in face of the reactions to the last depression, the fears of another one, the continuing popularity of welfare projects, and the persistent demands in some quarters for policies thought incompatible with the maintenance of that system. At the same time, of course, it is a testimony to continuing business influence and vitality. This ties in with the Cold War, in that the feelings of insecurity are intensified by the realization that "free enterprise" has been destroyed or put on the defensive in most of the rest of the world. This feeling of insecurity and unease, it should be emphasized, is not confined to business men, but is wide-spread throughout the society. This, I suggest, goes a very long way towards explaining the lack of opposition to the witch-hunt by people of influence. And lack of opposition is sufficient for the thriving of such a phenomenon. Among business men, of course, there is no uniform outlook in this respect, as in so many others. Opinion seems to range from the extremists who actively support Senator McCarthy and the Un-American Activities Committee, or its local counterparts, on the one hand, to those who have some distaste for the whole affair, on the other. The range is from the bitter die-hard anti-New-Deal Republicans to the more liberal Fair Deal Democrats (of whom Harriman is a fairly good example); but all are sufficiently anti-Communist and anti-Socialist not, so far at least, to have put up any determined resistance to the witch-hunt, however much they may have abstained from participating. Only, it seems to me, on the basis of some such hypothesis as that of business self-doubting, combined with business strength, can one explain the lack of opposition to the witch-hunt as well as the large element of hysteria discernible therein.

Finally, the witch-hunt must be seen against the background of the general tensions and insecurities present in American society today. Despite their continued assertion, the traditional values and standards of behaviour are constantly being questioned or flouted in many areas, and to a not insignificant degree. Most obviously, this state of affairs (which some sociologists now refer to as "anomy") is indicated by such things as the Kinsey Report (making all due allowances for overstatement and the smallness of the sample used in some cases) and the continuing revelations of political corruption. The point about these things is not simply that they are examples of ethical deviations, but that, while there are signs of a loosening in the hold on men's loyalties by the traditional standards, there are as yet no signs of the development of a new set of values to replace them. Accordingly, one finds in many quarters a more strident and aggressive proclamation of the old—which is much easier than trying either to find out why people ignore them (a course which may reveal an inadequacy in the values and not only in the "wrongdoers") or to amend the values. This last sentence may appear to contradict the earlier statement that the questioning process is very wide-spread. Certainly, the two attitudes described are contradictory, but, in the light of what is now known about human psychology, it does not follow that people may not hold both attitudes simultaneously. It follows only that inner conflict and tension will result—and that is the point I am concerned to make, by analogy, about American society today.

Mention has already been made of the unease regarding the economic system. There, even more obviously, one finds the absence of any agreed alternative, or of any alternative at all attractive to large numbers of Americans. And the economic doubts are potentially sharpened by the increasing rigidity in the economy and the relative diminution in opportunities for individual advancement, or, as some would say, by the closing of the frontier. That this is taking place, most economists and sociologists seem to agree. But the conflict between the ideals of free opportunity, social and economic advancement by merit and industry, and free competition, on the one hand, and the realities of increasing social economic rigidity, concentration of economic power, and limitation of competition (as being "unfair" or "cut-throat"), on the other, is masked and mitigated by the present arms-induced prosperity. However, if—as many seem now to be fearing—there should be another major recession, the conflicts may well become explosive.

To these conflicts must be added the perennial one revolving around the "Negro problem." That all these various types of tension and conflict, actual or potential, are by no means unconnected with the witch-hunt is indicated, I suggest, by the fact that amongst the most extreme hunters one finds those people who are also most anti-Negro, most anti-labour, and most vocally in favour of "morality" and "decency." In addition, and very important as a source of anxiety, is simply the fact of America's new role in the world. If only because of the close connection between the witch-hunt and the failure of American policy in China (the chances of its success being virtually nil), it is perhaps worth commenting that one of the great difficulties, for many Americans, arising out of their new world role, is that here is an area where the American tendency to look for once-for-all solutions of an almost "technological" nature is quite inappropriate, since any one country can control only a part of the situation, while foreign policy problems in general are usually very intractable at best.

The upshot of all the investigations, committees, hearings, "smear" campaigns, loyalty oaths and requirements, anti-sub-versive employment practices, passport regulations, denuncia-tions, informers, and so on, to which collectively I have referred as the witch-hunt, is to take the United States an appreciable degree along the road to a relatively polite and civilized form of totalitarianism. It is polite and civilized in that, as yet, no use has been made of concentration-camp brutality, "people's courts," or the rest of the less refined police-state techniques, and that it is still no crime to be a critic, although in effect it is a crime to be a Communist and in many cases it is unsafe to be too critical for fear of becoming unemployable in any but non-governmental and more or less manual jobs. And the United States has not progressed all the way along the road, in that, for example, highly "subversive" articles or books are still written, sometimes published, and occasionally read. But it seems to me impossible to deny that there exists a strong and well-organized campaign to limit the bounds of tolerable criticism very severely, and that this campaign is meeting with a great deal of success. It is true that this sort of thing has happened before—in the 1790's and early 1920's, for example—but on those occasions the persecution was either more sporadic and unorganized or faced with greater opposition, or both, than it is today. And, which is perhaps even more important, it did not take place against a background as well suited to the growth of an over-all political authoritarianism. For all the factors I discussed earlier in trying to account for the witch-hunt, are factors that can throw up a totalitarian regime of some sort or other. The prospect is not rendered the less dangerous by the feeling one has in America, often remarked upon before, that the resort to violence is never far away.

To let the matter rest there, however, is falsely to portray my impressions of the country as a whole. It is often pointed out that, politically, there are two Americas (at least): the one tending to be intolerant, impatient of reform, restrictive, and narrow in outlook, grossly materialist, Republican rather than Democratic (to use the modern conservative terminology), and clinging grimly to its privileges; and the other tolerant, reformist, imaginative, idealist, Democratic, liberal and humane. In varying forms, and to varying extents, the two Americas have struggled for ascendancy at least since the time of Hamilton and Jefferson. It is the second that has kept seeking "the promise of American life," never content to accept what seems unjust or unfair, while the first has tended rather to regard the promise as having been fulfilled by the Founding Fathers when they framed a Constitution satisfactory to the propertied interests. And it is the second that is under fire and on the defensive now, as yet unable to stem the flow of the witch-hunt being run on behalf of the extremists of the first. And it is because the first America seems to me to be dominant today, while the official spokesmen talk the language of the second, that I have devoted most of my space to discussing the present-day manifestations of "le noir" in America.

When all is said and done, the fact remains that the old liberal and revolutionary ideals are not dead—if they were, there would be no need for a witch-hunt—and it will not, probably, be easy to write them off completely. In one important respect, they have not yet even been seriously challenged—the social egalitarianism, the absence of that cap-touching servility and that separation of class by accent and manner which so mar the British scene, remains to delight the visitor and to point the way to a better life. And, with its size, its variations, and its contrasts, America still fascinates the observer. For these reasons among others, then, I have grown to like the country. So, I repeat, I hope I am wrong while fearing that I am right—not only because what happens in America must affect what happens in Britain and elsewhere, but also because I now care a great deal about what happens to Americans.   G. C. M., 1950

SOCIALISM ?⤳ I was interested to observe the reaction of Americans to the word "Socialism." Among the people I met it was usually regarded as something not even to be thought of, and certainly, if considered at all, to be contemplated with horror. Yet very few people, even university students, appeared to have a clear understanding of the meaning of this unspeakable word. Often a scheme which might be labelled "Socialistic" might be given some thought and found to have some merit, if mentioned without the label, but the word "Socialism" can be almost guaranteed to evoke a highly emotional reaction. My particular interest was in obtaining opinions on the much discussed subject of "socialized medicine." The term is unfortunate, for the word "socialized" immediately elicits a reaction of fear and revulsion in many. The propaganda of the American Medical Association has been successful in convincing a great many people that the National Health Service has been a dismal failure in Britain and hence a similar scheme would have no chance of succeeding in the United States. Many who favour extension of health services provided out of taxation hesitate to support it because of the fear of Federal interference in State affairs. The only people I met who were wholeheartedly in favour of a comprehensive health service provided by the government were social workers and public health nurses, who really know what ill health means to people in the lower income groups, and a dean of a medical school who had had considerable public health experience.

I had to learn a great deal about the United States before I could understand attitudes such as those I have mentioned. It seemed plain to me that there has been a steady trend towards government responsibility in many aspects of life where the welfare of the people as a whole is involved—in conservation and use of natural resources, in education, health, and social security generally. Then why are so many people apparently unwilling to accept this trend and resistant to further developments? After spending most of my life in New Zealand, where the government has always been expected to take this kind of responsibility, and where civil servants have continued in office and have been little affected by changes of government, I found the American mistrust of government, particularly central government and officialdom, difficult to comprehend.   A. M. R., 1952

NATIONALIZATION &» I believe that slowly but surely the country is being awakened from what has been a very pleasant dream. Despite the astonishingly high standard of living, people are beginning to realize that they can no longer afford to crop the land until it will crop no more and then seek pastures new; or to pump the water from the ground until they can no longer reach it; or to devastate their forests without replanting. Conservation was obviously an unknown word in America for many generations, but one hears it quite frequently today. And I believe that for all the vociferous complaints of the commercial world against Government controls and of the professional classes against the New Deal policies, these have come to stay. Resources will have to be conserved and developed for the good of all and private enterprise will have to be restrained, at least to some extent, so that a few individuals shall not gain their selfish ends at the expense of the community at large. I have found that most Americans still think far more in terms of their own community than of their State or of the nation as a whole—at any rate in domestic affairs—but just as they are being forced as a nation to realize their interest in and dependence on the rest of the world, so do I believe that they are being forced, within the nation, to realize the increasing dependence of one community on another and of one State on another in the modern age.

There are still enormous resources in the United States, and private enterprise has still a big part to play in developing them. But the financing of some of this development has been and still is beyond the capacity of any private or local community undertaking and the development itself, is, in many cases, of such wide public concern that I can see no alternative to a further expansion of Government activity and influence in certain fields. Many Americans have asked me (in sympathetic tones) about "nationalization" in Britain and I have countered by pointing to the Tennessee Valley Authority, the Bureau of Reclamation activities in the West, and the responsibility of the Corps of Engineers of the Army for all navigable harbours and rivers and for flood control works in the whole of the United States. There seems to me to be little difference between these and nationalized railways or harbours—and the Corps of Engineers has been responsible for harbours and rivers for many years.

Perhaps the United States thought of nationalization first! I must admit that, paradoxically, I myself have better appreciated the necessity for some form of governmental control in certain fields since I came to America than I did before I left Britain, though I still believe that what has to be found is a means of preventing excess of control from stifling private initiative and enterprise.

Various expedients have already been tried in the States. The Federal Government tries, as far as possible, to avoid having any part in the retail selling of electric power, and the whole of the power from some of the large dams in the West is sold to private power companies for distribution when it leaves the dam power stations; whilst in at least one case private companies actually operate the generators at the dam power station. Yet the control of water at the dam remains in Government hands, in order to safeguard the irrigation interests and to control floods. The Port of New York Authority is a self-supporting, non-profit-making authority representing the interests of two States and yet is able to finance new projects through public bond issues, repayable, both as to interest and capital, from tolls or other charges levied on the public. The control of and responsibility for all roads is shared by the States and the Federal Government—yet where a public benefit will result private companies are allowed to finance and build turnpike roads and large bridges and to levy tolls. The future development of nationalization in the United States will, I believe, be worth watching.   W. G. H., 1951

FEDERALISM ɞ✷ Many Americans who recommend federalism for Europe do not yet understand the, by comparison, tiny sacrifice of sovereignty required by membership in the United Nations.
                                                        A. P. S., 1952

CITY POLITICS ɞ✷ In Boston there was an election in which the notorious Curley machine, now in decay, was challenged by a "good government" organization known as the New Boston Committee. This type of organization is very common in American cities, and to discover what sort of animal it was I joined its ranks as a canvasser. The Committee, a group of well-meaning political amateurs running a completely honest campaign and relying almost entirely on voluntary workers, was able to win a majority in the City Council at its first election. It was a convincing demonstration of the advantages that can accrue from a fluid party system, but at the same time it seemed very clear to me that the Committee, which was bound together by no principle other than hostility to "the machine," was destined either to fall quickly into disunity or else to develop into a machine itself. In American cities the need for reform is intermittent but never-ending.   A. H. B., 1952

COUNTY POLITICS ɞ✷ The county seat has still a long future, I consider, as the mainstay of party organization in each State as a whole. It helps to do for the American party what the local branch (not governmental) of the British party does: it keeps together a nucleus of support between elections, provides a focus for party discussion and loyalty, and keeps the party leaders in the public eye. It does all this by methods which are, of course, comparatively unknown and certainly unsanctioned in Britain but which are integral to the American system: basically, the apportionment of county employment among supporters of the party in the majority. Any criticism of that feature of American local government (and indeed State and Federal government) which most often comes under fire—the elective nature of so many jobs which many Americans and all British commentators think might better, in this age, be appointive—must take into account the distinct possibility that if they ceased to be elective and so at the legal disposal of the party leader, they might be at his disposal by illegitimate and so even more objectionable means. A party system anywhere performs a controlling and co-ordinating function over organs of government otherwise disparate and centrifugal in tendency; it also will usually help to polarize issues, and thus render them more easily assimilable to the voter in the democratic process. Apart from any question of interests or jobs, therefore, a party system may be necessary to a system of government such as ours. Now the backbone of a State party organization, from sheer numbers, is not the city hall but the county hall machine. Short of a genuine disappearance of parties from the scene, there will be some such organization; and such a convenient locus as the county hall will not be given up by the mere institution of appointive offices or a civil service system. The question of which method is more efficient for the discharge of the official's duties is something of an "unreal" one, in the sense that it is hardly the true ground of battle. The propaganda war has been waged, as it almost always has to be, on a false front.   A. D., 1952

T.V.A. ࣿ To a geographer the real point of interest lies in the sphere of regional planning. The T.V.A.'s charter authorizes it to enter this field (Articles 22 and 23), and it must be said that most of the publicity issued by the Authority has been designed to create an impression that it was, in fact, a regional planning agency, transforming the whole of life within the Valley. Now, as soon as it makes these claims within the wider sphere, instead of confining its assertions to the narrower fields of flood control and power, it inevitably encounters heavy criticism. There are plenty of people who can point to aspects of Tennessee life which have *not* been improved by the coming of the T.V.A. But these criticisms would never have been launched if the T.V.A. had not set itself up to be a super life-changer when in fact it was nothing of the sort.

From documents examined by me in the T.V.A. library at Knoxville, Tennessee, it appears quite clear that Congress granted powers of regional planning without any consideration of what might be involved therein. These powers were granted "almost by accident," and the question (which the directors of the Authority were unable to answer) was whether their powers would be interpreted by Congress as spearheading an experiment in national planning. In the event, Congress does not appear to have given a second thought to the matter.

It thus came about that the T.V.A. became possessed of powers which had never been elaborated as part of a formal policy, which if exercised would undoubtedly bring the Authority into collision with other planning agencies, and which, as late as January, 1938, were still an enigma to the T.V.A.'s "Regional Planning Council." A document of that date shows the Council entirely ignorant of its terms of reference and still seeking an elaboration of the charter.

In point of fact, from 1938 onwards, regional planning as such was quietly dropped from among the tasks fulfilled by the T.V.A. I came across a number of regional surveys of that date which had never been carried through and of which the present staffs were in ignorance. Congress did not follow up with the "experiment in national planning," and the regional planning staff of the Authority was switched to other business. But all this time the publicity machine continued to paint a picture of a region transformed by planning and the critics continued to carp. Regional planning in a formal sense has never been carried out by

POLITICS   151

the T.V.A. It has planned dams and power lines, and, in my
opinion, has done creditable work. It has infiltrated into the field
of agriculture and helped matters there. But in regional planning
it has taught America nothing (which is profoundly to be deplored) because there has been no regional plan. Consequently
America faces, in the Missouri Valley, the Columbia Basin, the
Central Valley of California, and elsewhere, identical problems
of regional development without the benefit of any conclusive
lessons learned in the costly school on the Tennessee.

J. H. P., 1950

LOCAL AUTONOMY ੨ Centralization is a thing that in England
we tend to regard as an inevitable process (whether we like it
or not) which we can see steadily at work in our history for the
last thousand years. There is no such attitude in the United
States. It is common knowledge that the Federal Government
in the last twenty years has concerned itself in many matters
formerly regarded as outside its province. But there is an almost
universal feeling that this is wrong. The traditional attitude
(based on the historic fact that the local community came before
the State and the State before the Federal Government) is still
the general attitude today.

Similar, though perhaps not quite so intense, is the feeling
that the State governments should leave the local authorities to
manage their own affairs with the minimum of interference. In
fact, in many American cities, not only the Federal but the State
government seems very far away from City Hall.

Thus, in spite of the superficial standardization of the American scene (which most people seem not to dislike) and in spite of
the fact that every technical advance inevitably reduces differences and distances, there is a strong civic spirit which is more
than a sentimental attachment to the native place or an artificial
creation of the local Chamber of Commerce. It is rather a rea-
soned conviction that the local government and its independence

is an essential element in the balance of powers in which Americans see the safeguard of their liberties. Some aspects of local government seem odd to a visitor. It is strange to find the Town Clerk and the City Treasurer (Detroit) elected by the citizens and fighting an opposed election. But the sentiment itself is basically wholesome and admirable. It is a feature of American life which can be appreciated only on the spot (it does not get much attention from Hollywood) and it is one of the rewards of travel to have experienced it.   H. J. R., 1952

Religion

THE CHURCHES AND LOYALTY ⧼⧽ The energy, enthusiasm, resources, and efficiency of the American churches impressed me tremendously. The Briton can only sigh with envy when he sees much of this. There is no need for statistics to show that the influence and strength of the churches is growing daily; although it is interesting to learn from the statistics that the Protestant churches are growing slightly more rapidly (in numbers at any rate) than the Roman Catholic. The press, and day-to-day impressions, tend, I think, to suggest the opposite. More impressive than figures, and more impressive even than the massive physical resources which the churches now command for worship, education, and other activities, is the conclusion I formed almost everywhere that people's minds are open to what the churches have to say. If I add the comment that the churches' opportunity seems to be greater in some ways than they have yet realized, I should have to qualify it by saying that this is only one man's opinion based on very inadequate experience, and further that if this is true in America it is far more true in Britain; in Britain the churches' opportunity may be less obvious, but I am also convinced that both in thought and action they are far from doing enough to grasp it.

In this year of an American Presidential election and of a British coronation—events which stress many of the contrasts between America and Britain in the whole spiritual and political complex which makes up these nations' life—certain broad tendencies seemed to me to stand out.

In Britain, as Reinhold Niebuhr pointed out in an article at coronation time, the Crown is a symbol of the unity which underlies all political differences. As a symbol, high and lifted up above politics, it is deeply satisfying because it has a full, personal content; but when this is allied to the Englishman's comfortable sense of the permanence of his own institutions and their God-given stability, the result can be, and is, a kind of self-satisfaction which is very hard to break because it comes so near to the genuine demands of loyalty. In a sense, Englishmen (but not Scots, at least to the same extent) have solved the problem of loyalty too well. A courageous church in Britain must see that this is so, and must prescribe a remedy which will shake some of the self-satisfactions, as well as take account of the subconscious and conscious dissatisfactions which do exist.

In America, on the other hand, it seems to me manifest that the problem of loyalty is acute, at least on the superficial level. It may be that deeper down the elements of a stable solution are no less present than they are in Britain; but the solution is of a different kind. The symbols of loyalty in America are wholly political, and not in any explicit sense religious. This means that in one way the churches' task is easier; it is not necessary for the churches always to bear in mind their official political status when they make pronouncements that have political repercussions, for they have no such status. But in another way it makes their situation harder, for the political loyalty of the churches is not a *datum* (as it is in a certain sense in Britain) but a *desideratum;* and so they have to tread a narrow path between the necessary function of criticism and the appearance of disloyalty on a purely political level. The problem of loyalty is acute in America, or so it seems to me, because the content of the symbols of loyalty is changing and uncertain; this obviously applies to extrinsic symbols like the flag, which symbolize whatever is held to be the American idea by the contemporary generation. But it applies also to something so apparently specific as the Declaration of Independence or the Constitution; for after all there are many interpretations, when it comes to practice, of the principles therein contained. When the symbol is fixed, the content must change; when the symbol changes (as it does in a certain way with the British symbols) the content can in a strange way remain fixed.

It seems to me that it is just here, in this problem of loyalty, that the churches in America have a most important contribution to make. For loyalty, as Josiah Royce of Harvard insisted and as the present-day French existentialists among others are again discovering, is essentially a religious concept. The churches in America have already made some strong (and courageous) statements about certain tendencies in American politics which they consider dangerous; but it is of a rather more fundamental re-examination of what loyalty is that I am thinking. I am not suggesting that America should move, or is moving, towards a closer association of church and state, although there are indications that in certain ways this may be happening, but I am simply suggesting that this problem of loyalty should be thoroughly re-examined at all levels.   R. A. S. B., 1953

SPIRITUAL NEEDS ?? I felt that many Americans who have lost or never had a spiritual background for their beliefs are beginning to realize the necessity for it. . . . I did gain the impression that although most Americans do believe in high ethical and moral standards, they are not quite sure why they hold these beliefs and are therefore not prepared to fight for them. They seek to explain them on sociological grounds, but without any belief in absolute values of right or wrong they can never be certain where the dividing line should lie. As a people they have many virtues, but one of these—tolerance—seems to me to be carried beyond the limits of virtue, until it has almost become a vice. How else can one explain the extraordinary *laissez-faire* attitude of the average American to such things as corruption in public life, organized crime, or cheating in colleges, as exposed in recent months? My general impression was that most people feel that these things are wrong, but that they have not sufficient conviction to want to rise up and stamp them out. So they just shrug their shoulders—and tolerate them.

It is true that certain public men of high integrity and some sections of the press are trying to stir up public opinion against these things, but until the people themselves show that they will *not* tolerate them, Americans will never gain the respect and confidence of the world they seek to lead. Respect for their material achievements and confidence in their enormous productive power the world may have, but not the respect for their character and ideals and confidence in their integrity that is so essential to the friendship which I believe most Americans do earnestly desire from other nations. They must first crystallize their beliefs and find a solid basis for them, so that the rest of the world may know beyond any doubt where they are being led, and by what sort of people.

It is my conviction that only by a wide-spread renewal of belief in Christianity can this be achieved, and I was encouraged by the signs I saw that considerable efforts are being made in this direction. There are a great many practicing Christians in the States and I was greatly struck by the work that is being done by these people and by the churches themselves to provide religious instruction for the young people. Yet I was distressed to see what obstacles they have to overcome. Surely the authors of the Constitution would turn in their graves if they knew that the words they wrote nearly two centuries ago, with the object of safeguarding religious freedom, are now being construed to mean that the people shall have freedom from religion? The absence of religious teaching in the schools is not, perhaps, of great consequence where the children have Christian parents, but it does mean that a great many of the younger generation, whose parents hold no such beliefs, must be growing up without any real knowledge of religion at all.

I believe that the United States, together with the British peoples, can give the world the moral leadership it so badly needs. There are already signs of revolt against the evil in their midst—but the States have been thrust into their position of leadership so suddenly that there is no time to lose, if they are to persuade the peoples of the world that the "American way of life" is not only materially but also spiritually far higher than that which Russian Communism can give them.

W. G. H., 1951

CHURCH-GOING ࿎ Does the American, brought up to believe that attendance at church is a desirable trait, merely put this belief into action with his usual thoroughness? Does he attend church because he finds a spiritual pick-me-up helpful after a week of keen business activity? Or does he go to worship God? I am inclined to the belief that while the swollen churches may give a false and magnified first impression of the religious fervour of the Americans, there is nevertheless a wide-spread religious sincerity. The multiplicity of cults and sects in America is a frequent target of criticism. False some of the "prophets" may be, and the followers of some of the extremist cults may be misguided in their enthusiasm, but there is something reassuring in this evidence of spiritual vigour in a nation so lavishly endowed materially.

J. D. R., 1951

CHURCH AND SOCIETY ࿎ On a Sunday, in most towns, the sidewalks are crowded with people either going to church or coming from it. Out of a population of around 157 millions, 120 millions are said to go to some church or other on Sundays. It would be naïve to conclude that 120 millions are therefore Christians.

Church-going, in America as elsewhere, may simply be a habit or a social convention. In the States it may be a rigorous application of the principle of equality driving people to conform to the group. It may be un-American to stay away from church. But when all that is said, this amazing fact cannot solely be ascribed to group sense or to the wish to mingle with the herd. Un-American to stay away from church? The background to this statement is my impression that there is a too easy identification of the American way of life with Christianity. In practically all the churches, irrespective of denomination, the Stars and Stripes and the Church Flag stand opposite to each other in the chancel. This is a kind of symbol of what I mean. It is a very great question to ask whether Americans are Americans first and Christians second, but one wonders if the churches are playing a sufficiently active role as critic of society when Governor Stevenson's remark about Communism could be regarded as something quite novel and surprising. I refer to the remark, "When we [in the U.S.A.] think of Communism we think of what we have to lose; when they [the Asiatics] think of it they think of what they are to gain."

Yet I would not presume to judge the American churches solely on their attitude to Communism. The dominant impression was along quite different lines. I had started off thinking specifically of the American churches—approaching them, as it were, critically and objectively. The dominant impression, at the end, was not of the American churches but of the world church. . . . I had been led to this view by the prayers and some of the sermons I had heard, by talks with church folk up and down the country—and above all by the reception given to me at Union Seminary and the interest and questioning about the Church of Scotland and its tradition. The consciousness of their membership of the world church, however, has to become a great deal more articulate throughout the various denominations, and there is much to be learned from the hard experiences of other churches in Europe. As this takes place, the American churches may come to realize the dangerous false security of "fashionable Christianity" and have the courage to occupy a less comfortable but more realistic position—in terms of the Gospel —in society.   D. G., 1951

Police

AMERICAN POLICE SYSTEMS ᘓᔌ The States watch jealously that the Federal Government exercises no powers other than those specifically conferred upon it, and regard themselves as sovereign powers in all other respects; to take a small instance, the traffic laws vary from State to State, and the regulations about licensing motor-cars and about such matters as whether a right turn is permitted on a red signal depend on the law in force in the particular State. Some of the States, such as Pennsylvania and Massachusetts, call themselves "Commonwealths," and it is to be remembered that in population and wealth some of the States are quite as large as independent countries in other parts of the world. But just as the States watch that the Federal Government does not usurp too much power, so do the smaller local government areas within the State resist the assumption of too much power by the State; and one of the marks of authority which a unit of local government, however small, will wish to retain is the police power. It is doubtful if there is any other country where local autonomy in police management has been carried to such lengths.

On each step of the ladder of government, from the village up through the township to the city, the State, and the Federal Government, there is likely to be a police agency. But the picture is even more complicated than that. A second dimension, as it were, is introduced by the fact that at each of these levels there are likely to be enforcement agencies created for special and limited services. . . .

A village might well have its own marshal and be situated within a township which has its own constable, which in its turn

is situated in a county which has its own sheriff's organization,
which in its turn is in a State with its own State police force.
If a crime were committed the aggrieved citizen could complain
to any of the four—constable, marshal, sheriff, or State trooper—
all of whom have jurisdiction.

In Oakland County, Michigan, for instance, the State police
patrol the highway; the sheriff is responsible for policing the
county; the county prosecutor has his own staff of investigators;
each of the twenty-five townships into which the county is di-
vided has a constable; three of these townships also have their
own police departments; there are ten villages which have their
own marshals; and there are fourteen cities which have their
own police departments. Within a fifteen-mile radius of Boston
Common there are forty cities and towns, each with its own
police system, and the entire area is criss-crossed by the parkway
patrols of the Metropolitan District Commission. Within a fifty-
mile radius of Chicago there are 350 police forces—municipal,
county, and State. In a street in, say, Los Angeles there might
at any one time be a patrol car of the State highway patrol passing through; a sheriff's county car crossing through the city to
reach one of the islands of territory policed by the county; an
ordinary Los Angeles Police Department patrol car; a Los
Angeles accident investigation car on its way to a street accident; a patrol car of the juvenile department of the city police;
and an F.B.I. car directed by radio to the scene of a bank robbery—which incidentally might, or might not, prove to be a
Federal offence. . . .

The police in the U.S.A. have always lived under the shadow
of politics, and the influence of politics in police administration
remains today of the first importance. It is not merely that some
of the police chiefs themselves—particularly the sheriffs—are
elected by the people and run at the elections on a party ticket;
it means that in many areas members of a police force look to
the politicians for assistance in getting themselves appointed to

the force, in getting promotion, in avoiding or securing transfer, or in avoiding disciplinary action; and the politician is apt to expect some return for favours conferred. In the cities, the mayor, who is an elected officer, is very much more powerful than the mayor of an English town, and he may well be able to intervene with considerable effect in the organization and running of the city police department. In recent years, it has become more common for the rank and file of a police department to be appointed on Civil Service conditions (that is, for them to hold a permanent, pensionable appointment), but the members of Civil Service departments are themselves not immune from the suggestions and influences of politicians. In any event, it is still normal for the *head* of the police department to be appointed by the party in power without any security of tenure and for a change to be made when there is a change of administration. The fact that Mr. J. Edgar Hoover has retained his office as Director of the Federal Bureau of Investigation through the regimes of four presidents is regarded as a phenomenon. . . .

The F.B.I., unlike the other Federal agencies, is not on Civil Service. Its members can be dismissed at pleasure, and the inefficient cannot expect to stay very long. It dates back to 1908, its first responsibilities having been in effect limited to the suppression of the white slave traffic. In 1924 Mr. J. Edgar Hoover became Director, and the work and the size of the Bureau have since then been steadily increased as new acts of Congress have created new Federal offences—kidnapping, taking a stolen car across a State frontier, taking a woman across a State frontier for immoral purposes, and so on. During the war the Bureau had a general responsibility for co-ordinating security matters; and in some of the field offices I visited, security questions constituted more than half the work—including not only ordinary security matters such as watching Communist activities, but also such matters as checking the records of prospective

Government employees. Without being disrespectful to the Bureau, one of its most important achievements lies in the impression it has given to the public of its efficiency, and in what it has done to enlist public sympathy for the forces of law and order and to improve the status of the police officer. . . .

A candidate for appointment as a Special Agent in the Federal Bureau of Investigation (there are no Ordinary Agents) must be either a lawyer or an accountant—a condition which gives some indication of the work expected of Special Agents. They are not normally engaged in pursuing violent gangsters and murderers. They are trained in the use of firearms and have to keep in practice, and they sometimes run across the more violent criminals, for instance when investigating the robbery of a Federal bank; but on the whole the more spectacular crimes are usually State offences, and the long list of Federal crimes is made up for the most part of crimes which do not normally involve violence. A Special Agent is more likely to be concerned with clearing up a motor-car theft, or a complicated fraud, or checking the record of an applicant for employment at an atomic bomb factory, than with chasing an armed murderer. . . .

The Texas Rangers (which still function as a small detective force) were perhaps the first of the State police forces, but originally they were really a border patrol. Early State police forces with limited functions were set up in Massachusetts and Connecticut, but the history of the modern State police dates from 1905, when a force was set up in Pennsylvania with the conscious intention of using it as a general executive arm for the State. . . . It now has a strength of about 1,600, being the biggest of the State police forces; the troopers do the whole of their patrolling by car and are primarily, but by no means exclusively, concerned with traffic regulations. Pennsylvania set a fashion. New York, Michigan, West Virginia, Maryland, and, quite recently, Vermont, are among the states which have followed, in substance, the example set by Pennsylvania. Almost half the States now have State police forces with full police powers. The better State police forces, thanks to their recent creation, their State-wide responsibilities, and the fact that on the whole their commanders have been able men, have managed to keep much clearer of politics than the ordinary city force. They have set a high standard of entrance qualifications, and although the salary they now offer is usually no higher than that in the bigger city forces, they have succeeded in attracting a high type of recruit and apparently have no difficulty in securing an abundance of well-educated and suitable candidates—some of them from city police forces who are prepared to lose their city service on transfer. From the start, they have placed emphasis on training, and as a result the State trooper in the better forces is normally a well-trained, efficient, and courteous officer with a high standard of responsibility and pride in the organization of which he is a member. . . .

The circumstances of the sheriff's appointment mean that he need have no training in or particular qualifications for police work, and he may not remain in office long enough to acquire any great fund of experience and knowledge. In some areas his staff is permanent, but in most places the deputies are appointed by the sheriff of the day, and there may therefore be a complete change when there is a change of sheriff. There are exceptions to this gloomy picture, particularly in the West, where the sheriff is a much more thriving and vigorous institution than he is in the East. . . .

Traffic is a major concern of the police in the United States. In California, with a population of ten millions, there are four million registered motor-cars, double the number in Great Britain, and there are several hundred thousands from other States also in California at any one time. This is the extreme example, but everywhere the motor-car is accepted as the normal means of conveyance. This affects police work in a number of ways. In the first place, the great volume of traffic calls for elaborate

methods of control and enforcement of traffic regulations; traffic
is certainly as important an aspect of police work as the prevention and detection of crime. In many States there is a highway patrol which is concerned solely with traffic and not
with crime in the ordinary sense; and where there is a State
police force, traffic is its dominant concern. Indeed, all forces,
whatever their other interests, must put traffic in the forefront
of their activities. In this field the American police are facing
problems (and are evolving techniques to cope with them) which
are on a scale much greater than anything our police are likely
to meet with for some years to come. . . .

At present, the police in the United States have a difficult
job to do, both in the matter of crime detection and prevention
and in the control of traffic; and on the whole they are so organized as to make this difficult task still more difficult.

P. A., 1949

EVASION OF LAWS ➜ It is still fair to say, I think, that a large
proportion of the citizens lack a high instinct for order and a
sense of the dignity of obedience to restraint which is demanded
for the common good. The citizens themselves often do not want
strict law enforcement; they may justify this by appealing to
the American concept of personal liberty, but as Mr. Bruce Smith
has pointed out, in this context the concept of personal liberty
only too often means a belief that the police should not do anything about the illegal activity with which the citizen in question
may be concerned, and that if he should be caught, then it ought
to be possible for the authorities to be "fixed". . . .

There are many sumptuary laws (of which prohibition was an
outstanding example) which attempt to regulate the personal
habits and morals of the citizens; which create offences which
are not condemned by public opinion; which are enforced rarely,
or in a capricious manner, according to the feelings of the prosecutor holding office at the time; and which contrast strangely

with the American's emphasis that his country is the great stronghold of individual rights and intolerance of needless authority. The existence of these laws, and the capriciousness of their enforcement, tend to make more difficult the general problem of law enforcement; but the average member of a State legislature does not yet seem to have learned that a problem is not removed merely by passing a law which condemns it but does not include any effective sanctions against it. In New Orleans it used to be an offence to sell tobacco on Sundays. The tobacco stalls therefore concealed themselves behind green curtains, which had the dual effect of making some gesture to the law and of advertising the whereabouts of the stands.   P. A., 1949

MURDER! ᘒ In the city of Houston, Texas, with a population of 600,000, the number of murders in a year is about the same as the number for the whole of England and Wales.   P. A., 1949

Road Traffic

THE AUTOMOBILE AGE (1) ᘒ Probably the most potent influence on the American citizen is the automobile, itself a by-product of American industrial success. . . .

The numbers in use are worth recalling in comparison with other countries. In 1950, there were 40,000,000 automobiles in the United States for a population of about 150,000,000 people, about one for every four persons; in Los Angeles, there was one automobile for every 1.5 persons. The country with the next largest number of automobiles was Great Britain with 2,300,000 for a population of 50,000,000 people, that is, about one car for every twenty people. . . .

The automobile has made its mark on the landscape in the shape of service stations, motels, restaurants, and curio shops, most of them giving good service to the traveller, but nearly all having glaring advertisements, extending for miles and spoiling the view at almost every beauty spot visible from the highway. The automobile, too, is responsible for keeping the excellent national parks in existence. All these things are the outward and visible signs of the reign of the automobile, which must be remembered when attempting comparisons of the United States with any other country; they are possibly of little spiritual significance. The recreational habits of the whole American people are obviously affected. Walking has gone out of fashion to such an extent that on the outskirts of towns there are usually no footpaths for pedestrians; and rural roads never have any. It appeared that only in the greatest of cities, such as New York or Washington, is walking still practiced. I believe this represents a loss more serious than the mere loss of a healthy exercise. A long walk provides an excellent opportunity for straightening out mental difficulties.

The American is a confirmed automobilist, as opposed to the Briton, who is often an anti-motoring pedestrian, or a cyclist. There is therefore a different attitude towards the vehicle, towards safety on the roads, and towards the transportation system of the country. The American driver is almost part of "the American way of life"—something almost sacred. This attitude may perhaps influence the trend of researches on road safety, which tend to concentrate on the investigation of vehicle accidents rather than pedestrian accidents, and on methods of fitting the road to the vehicle, rather than vice versa. It is possible to get new street lighting only on traffic routes for the benefit of vehicle drivers, not in residential areas. The make and size of the automobile and the number owned are signs of social status, and replace our English equivalents, the size of house, the kind of accent, and the time one has dinner. It would be interesting to investigate how far the hire-purchase payments on automobiles are responsible for the energy with which many Americans devote themselves to the business of making money.   G. G., 1952

THE AUTOMOBILE AGE (2) ह‍ So many cars. This was my first impression. It seemed to symbolize the United States, or at least a certain important aspect of it that I was to get to know better

in Chicago. Each individual life sealed off in its own metal com-
partment, speeding along the highway with an appearance of
effortlessness but really involving an immense, even if habitual,
sense of responsibility, of skill in manoeuvre. The cars passed,
checked speed, occasionally halted, hooted anxiously, set off
again. The spectacle was fascinating and rather disquieting.

                                                    J. F. M., 1951

Business and Labour

THE SOCIAL ROLE OF THE BUSINESS MAN ᢒᢌ To a very large extent, it is to the business man that is reserved that social leadership which, in Britain, has been shared more widely with the
aristocracy, the "county" families, the retired government servant (particularly the retired colonial ruler), and the senior
military officer as well as, in much lesser degree, the preacher
and the teacher; to which list, in recent years, must be added
the trade union leader. Allied to the business man is the lawyer;
but since, traditionally, the lawyer has been hardly distinguish-
able (in outlook) from the business man (his chief "employer,"
after all) no special consideration need be given him here. This
social ascendancy manifests itself clearly in many community
associations and activities, in the composition of the boards of
trustees of universities and schools, and, especially at times of
mobilization like these, in appointments to key government positions. On closer examination, too, it appears, very naturally, that
the most important positions are held by, or on the sufferance of,
the most important business men—the representatives of the major
corporations. This is not to overlook the changes which have
taken place in the last twenty years—the increase in numbers and
strength of organized labour, the expanded jurisdiction and activities of government, welfare legislation, and the extent to which
government service (but not politics) has become a more "respectable" career for the able and ambitious, to name some of
the most important. On the contrary, these changes make the posi-

tion of the business man all the more remarkable. Nor should it be forgotten that during these same two decades, the increasing concentration of control within the economy has continued, as has the expanding wealth of the larger corporations, taxes notwithstanding.

Perhaps even more striking to the foreign observer, however, is the degree to which business ways of thinking, business standards of judgment are accepted throughout the society. The New Deal, at its most radical, never officially questioned the bases of the economic system, but rather was concerned to safeguard them by "civilizing" business; labour also stands for "free enterprise" and accepts most of the traditional ideology of success and prosperity and so on. What this amounts to is simply that business in America, and especially the hundred or so largest corporations, still possesses tremendous power as well as vitality. This power is economic most obviously, increasingly political (i.e., directly political rather than indirectly by corrupt means as in the past) as the merging of government and business proceeds, and social in some degree; and there is the danger that it will yet more consciously and deliberately become a power over men's minds as "public relations" techniques are still further refined and as the need increases. Coming from Labour Britain, one is particularly struck by the relative openness and, almost, the immunity (except from criticism at election time) of American business power. This probably reflects popular pride in the undoubted achievements and benefits of American capitalism, as well as distrust. For there is distrust of and even, since the Great Depression, a suggestion of a challenge to the business man, which is also an important part of the picture, and a part necessary to the understanding of the atmosphere today.

G. C. M., 1950

BUSINESS AS SPORT ?∾ Undoubtedly America is a business civilization in many ways. As there is little that corresponds to a hereditary aristocracy in the European sense, the successful business man stands very high in the social scale. Far greater prestige attaches to such a figure than to a university professor. The achievement of wealth through one's own efforts is the ideal, and other pursuits are thought inferior. Where the young man just down from Oxford or Cambridge regards (or pretends to regard) a business career with slight aversion, the majority of graduates from Yale and Harvard have no doubt that their future lies in some business enterprise, though they may further gird themselves for the fray at the Yale Law or Harvard Business Schools. The aphorism that in America "sport is a business, and business a sport," is truer than most. In business fortune may be found, absorbing interest, and the esteem of one's neighbours. Business is a national enthusiasm; the undergraduate "heelers" in the universities handle their various errands with an energy and competence quite foreign to their English counterparts, whether they be selling Christmas cards and toothpaste, or negotiating contracts for the Student Pressing Agency. One American boy who had visited Oxford told me he saw no opportunities for the go-ahead young man there. When I suggested that study ought to be the concern of the student he replied, "Yes, but not *all* the time. How can you ever learn to *run* anything at Oxford?" He was not a stupid boy, nor an unusual undergraduate here. He simply liked activity, and thought activity in business the most interesting occupation. Why be ashamed of wanting to do things well, to live well and buy nice clothes for a pretty wife, who would keep her looks ten years longer than the women he had seen in England? Why was pursuing wealth worse than pursuing foxes? You could eat with money, but you couldn't eat a fox. Business in short, *was* a sport for him, and is for many Americans. And, as D. W. Brogan and others have noted, the accumulation of wealth does not usually lead to avarice; when the American has acquired enough, he begins to give his money away to funds, to hospitals, to political parties, to his Alma Mater. The excitement lies ulti-

mately not in the hoarding of wealth, but in the getting, spending, and donating of it.   M. F. C., 1949

PUBLIC RELATIONS ❧ Faith in publicity is deep-rooted in the
American character, and it is not surprising that a nation which
is spending some 3,000 to 4,000 million dollars a year on advertising should believe that the methods that have been so effective
in selling toothpaste and soft drinks should also be effective for
selling attitudes and ideas.

First as "press-agentry," then as "publicity," now more grandi-
osely as "public relations," high-powered publicity is no novelty
on the American scene. Press agents flourished in the 19th century, and the term "public relations" began to be used before
the First World War. As an aftermath of the recent war and as
a facet of the post-war boom, the last few years have, however,
seen a striking increase in the various and sometimes odd activities that go under the name of public relations. These activities
include not only straight publicity, but barely disguised propaganda and lobbying, supposedly scientific advice on the shaping of
policy to conform to mass opinion and contrariwise on the moulding of mass opinion to conform to policy, and a whole host of
specialties such as "labour relations," "stockholder relations,"
"alumni relations," ad infinitum. "Watch Out: Human Problems
Ahead," advertised one of the best known and most flamboyant
public relations counsels in a full page of the *New York Times:*
"The Social Sciences can serve industry's human relationships
in the same way that physical sciences serve industry's technological progress." If the public relations man has bacon to sell, said
an unfriendly writer, "he makes use of the conditioned reflex;
he does not mention bacon at all, he manages a kind of vogue
for heartier breakfasts."

For the most part, however, public relations to the uninitiated
is synonymous with publicity, and in this sense it pervades
American institutions. Public relations directors or similarly des-

ignated employees are to be found not only in the big business corporations, but in universities (where they flourish remarkably), schools, trade unions, libraries, museums, churches, voluntary organizations, hospitals, and social welfare agencies, as well as in government. In some of these spheres their hold is as yet tenuous, but they are going ahead in every kind of organization which has a special interest in cultivating public support. That is logical enough, and the increased employment of technicians for duties which others would in any event have to do is merely a facet of the still growing specialization which characterizes the American society.

Natural exuberance as well as muddled thinking explains some of the more extravagant claims which are being made on behalf of the new profession. The establishment of the School of Public Relations at Boston University in 1947, one of the enthusiasts told the School, was "no less a milestone than the establishment of the schools of law, medicine, and engineering," and the President of the University claimed that it had transformed a "nondescript 'job' into a profession comparable with . . . the ministry, law, medicine and teaching." "Public relations," said a leading public relations counsel in a lecture at the school, "is founded upon the precepts of the Man who long ago, in the hills of Galilee, made religion understandable."

As the more percipient public relations leaders are aware, the future is, however, less assured than might at first sight appear. The testing time will come if there is a slump and budgets have to be stripped of all but essentials. Partly because of the nature of their activities, partly through their own fault, public relations practitioners enjoy singularly bad public relations. The public relations associations are disposed to blame the charlatans and crooks whom they would like to eliminate from the ranks of the aspiring profession. But the cause goes deeper than this. There is a natural suspicion of "fixers" and propagandists. It is felt that the mystery and the jargon with which some public relations people have surrounded themselves have often been adopted as covers for the nakedness underneath the impressive exterior.

J. A. R. P., 1948

NOTES ON "KNOW-HOW" 🙐 This expressive American word means any kind of technical skill, and includes technique, technology, applied science, and all the rest. They all deal with what can be reduced to a formula and put into a textbook—the generalized practical knowledge that knows nothing of human values, nor of the human purposes that lie behind its application. Although far from being confined to the mechanical arts, much of its terminology is derived from them by analogy. For example, in America one is surprised to learn of "workshops" where instead of bringing hammer, pincer, and nails, one comes armed with pencil and pad of paper to discuss some problem, let us say, of sociology around a table. Later we shall come to particular examples of know-how for securing the efficiency of organizations, teaching new skills, and effectively communicating ideas, all of which are far removed from mechanics proper.

America's great strength in regard to know-how does not lie so much in the quantity accumulated, although this is, of course, a factor, but rather in the following national characteristics:

1. Great confidence and verve in its use
2. Great ability to originate or adapt new forms of it for any and every practical purpose
3. What amounts to genius for imparting it widely through "extension"

and, perhaps most important of all:

4. The belief in America at her best that it is something to be used in furthering the welfare of mankind as a whole and so to be made freely available, rather than closely guarded as a source of power and advantage over others.

None of these characteristics in any way forms part of technology itself. They lie quite beyond it and are of another order. They arise from the values which Americans share, and spring from their history, traditions, and ideals. This sort of thing is more difficult to export than a case or two of textbooks.

When two sides possess much the same outlook and general way of life, there is no particular difficulty over the interchange of technical methods, and the whole thing can largely be left to the experts of that particular field. This is what in effect happened in the case of the Anglo-American productivity teams, all of whose reports tell a similar story. They gave the same technical reasons why American productivity is increasing at double the British rate: more mechanization, more power, more equipment in the U.S., and so on. But these are reasons, not explanations: they give the "how" but not the "why." The latter pointed to differences in outlook quite outside the scope of technological considerations. In the report "We Too Can Prosper," written for the British Productivity Council, the following key conclusion was reached: "To change that outlook requires not the knowledge of the techniques for prosperity—that is already there—but the will to prosper." So we see that even in an apparently straightforward case like this it is the human element on which all else turns.

How much more is this the case in the transmission of technical information to countries in which the cultural and economic differences are profound. All the easy assumption of broadly similar attitude and motivation breaks down hopelessly and the human problems are altogether more intractable. What these countries always want are certain aspects of technological civilization that strike them as desirable, without taking on the whole thing, still less losing their own way of life. But this is never possible. The fruits of technical development cannot be isolated in this way. Once the start is made, it is followed by progressive stages which end by breaking down the old way of life completely, with all the misery and demoralization involved in the collapse of old values and beliefs without substitution of effective new ones.

There is an excellent but extreme example of this in one of the Cornell University studies. The only implement of a community of Australian aborigines was a stone ax. Some well-meaning missionaries, hoping to make life easier for them, started distributing steel axes. It had quite the opposite effect. The annual migrations along trade routes designed to secure materials for the stone axes had been minutely governed by hierarchic custom and were the basis of the social organization. This fell to pieces when any youngster could get a far superior ax merely by going to the mission house. The effects on the community were disastrous. Fortunately, most other societies are tougher and more adaptable, but the story well illustrates the disruption and unforeseen consequences which the impact of Western technology inevitably causes.   F. P. C., 1953

UNIONS AND CAPITALISM ಶ್ಲ The labour movement in the U.S. is still basically content to act only as a pressure-group within the existing system as opposed to striking out as a political party with definite long-term political objectives. Union leaders continually join in the universal praise of free enterprise, and seem primarily concerned with obtaining a larger share of the proceeds. To put it another way—their ambitions shaped by the business world in which they operate, the unions are more concerned with increasing their power within a given industry, while maintaining the structure of ownership intact, than with endeavouring to alter the pattern of industrial and corporate ownership as a means to increasing labour's power and status within society as a whole. Along with this goes a general acceptance of the values and goals of industrial capitalism (efficiency, monetary rewards, work, success, and so on) and a sharing of the frequently limited and selfish aims of the industry in which the union operates, a sharing which is often encouraged by "enlightened" management policies of welfare and so on. It is true that union policies are such as to imply and necessitate many departures from the traditional notion of a free competitive economy, but these departures are not so much in the direction of Socialism as of a variety of corporate syndicalism, of a partnership of management and union leaders united against or to control the government and the consumer. This process has reached an advanced stage already in such industries as building (in many areas) and (in some ways) the New York garment trade. There is no reason at all why this should prove harmful to the interest of the controllers of big businesses in the long run—as some seem already to be realizing—whatever it might be to the interests of the community at large. I do not wish to imply that there are no elements of this in the British Trade Union movement, for there undoubtedly are; but it is not the sole, nor always the predominating, doctrine. One should also add that in many of the CIO unions, at least, there are sections which would prefer a more political role—but they are unlikely to win many converts so long as the present spell of prosperity and full employment lasts.

Although there is an old liberal reforming tradition in America, there is at the moment no real liberal movement. Further, there never has been one, in the sense of an organized movement continuing over a long period. Instead, there have been a series of protest movements, of which the most significant have originated among farmers, which have lasted not much longer than the period of economic depression which has set them off, or only until the policy has been taken over (usually in moderate form) by one of the major parties.

For this there would seem to be at least three reasons. First, all parties and all men talk in the language of the American Revolution and its liberal ideals, even if these symbols are manipulated for different purposes. Secondly, the traditional aims of European liberal parties—suffrage extension, the removal (in favour of the middle classes) of the legal barriers to social mobility and the other formal bulwarks of privilege, and the establishment of a "free" economy—all have seemed to be fulfilled in the United States for most people, at least, since the Civil War. And what is left to be done—trust-busting, the ending of racial discrimination, emphasis on civil rights, and so on—is in some cases not popular enough as a doctrine, in others not sufficiently distinctive to seem to necessitate a separate party, and in all cases hardly adds up to a coherent, significant, and sufficiently general program capable of serving as a sure guide for action on a wide front or in changing circumstances. All this is quite apart from the general causes leading to a world-wide decline in liberalism, of which one need only mention the failure of present-day liberals to cope with, or even recognize often, the role of power, other than state power, in political life.

Thirdly, the nature of American political parties with their decentralization, their doctrinal cross-breeding, and their failure to provide clear lines of responsibility in government, also militates against the establishment of a liberal party—and not even F.D.R. was able to liberalize the Democratic Party in any very extensive, or lasting, manner. As a result of this, and other, features of American politics, the isolated, disillusioned, and frustrated liberal is a typical figure of post-war America. He has nowhere to go, no significant group to join, and in many cases little or no hope for the future. His last chance for effective action seems to have passed with the demise and the Communist capture of the 1948 Progressive Party. Such groups as remain, like the ADA or ACLU, for all the useful work they do in individual cases of injustice, are little more than small pressure-groups whose chief function, only too often, is simply to give liberals some sort of feeling that they are "doing something." The relevance of this for labour is that, with little chance of obtaining a large accession of support from elsewhere, as is necessary for the successful launching of a third party or the taking over of an old one, even the politically minded union leaders must feel that they still have much more to gain by pressure-group activities.

G. C. M., 1950

INDUSTRIAL PSYCHOLOGY ⁊❧ In a country where the private or free enterprise system has competition and the profit motive is the spur to greater achievement, where government control and regulation are regarded by the business man as being synonymous with inefficiency and incompetence, and where natural resources and immigrant labour have in the past been exploited by some for the sake of quick profits, it is interesting to record a greater awareness of the human element as an important factor in the drive for increased productivity and a higher standard of living than has ever been apparent in the past. Employees are no longer a commodity to be used in the same way as a raw material in the manufacturing process but are becoming the centre of research, of investigation, and of co-operative experiment in an endeavour to give the employee full satisfaction at his job and with his prospects and, at the same time, obtain his participation in company policy and progress with pride in its achievements. With this growth in the awareness of the importance of the human element in industry goes the corresponding growth, at least in the larger corporations, of a feeling of moral responsibility for the effect of company changes and practices on the community in which they operate.   C. E. C., 1948

PROSPERITY—A LAYMAN'S VIEW ⁊❧ The elevator man at the Rockefeller Institute was never one to let his passengers ride in awkward silence. He always had something to tell or to ask, and after my ears became accustomed to the language of Brooklyn, I found my journeys from A to 6, or the reverse, were quite enjoyable. "Say, Doc, what does this?" he asked, and he showed the carload of medical authorities several patches of pimples on his face. These patches apparently had resisted all the proprietary creams. The authorities had little to suggest, however, and I thought no more about it. Then one morning some weeks later, he told us that he had cured the pimples himself and moreover the cure was really quite simple. He had just stopped eating steak every night for dinner!

I was in the land of good living indeed when our elevator man could eat steak regularly at well over a dollar per pound. Later I found out that he stayed in a very cheap apartment in order to live well, but nevertheless his diet, together with the long cigarette butts lying at all the bus stops, impressed me very strongly in my early days in New York that I had come to a land where shortages, rationing, and the watching of every penny hardly existed. As I moved around the United States, I saw that the vast majority of the people enjoys a standard of living very much higher than I had imagined in spite of my being mentally prepared for improved conditions.

Where does it come from? What makes this prosperity? Ask a shopkeeper in New York or a taxi-driver in Chicago; ask a student in Illinois or a farmer in Vermont. Four times out of five you will get the answer, "American private enterprise." In its broadest sense, this answer says that the prosperity is due to the boldness and the drive of the American individual in his undertakings, and taken thus it goes a long way towards the right answer. It ought to be interesting to set down a layman's observations on the great prosperity of the American people which will serve to expand this answer.

First on the list of factors contributing to prosperity come natural resources. In my travels, I saw vast fertile farm lands, powerful rivers, great supplies of natural gases, coal, sulphur, and other chemicals, the oil fields, timber forests, and rich metallic deposits. I was left in no doubt that the people of the United States are very fortunate indeed in their natural wealth.

However, without efficient harnessing and gathering of these resources, there would be no universal high standard of living. Both have been achieved by means of mechanization, and it is this that I place as the second factor leading to prosperity. The Americans have mechanized on an enormous scale, quite outstripping all others. This is due in part to the fact that mechanization for mass-production is an American idea. They were in at the start and have maintained their lead. The other reason is that the working man in the United States does not resist large-scale mechanization in the way workers sometimes do in other countries. The American sees expansion accompanying or following mechanization and he does not now seem to fear unemployment as a result of the advance of the machine. He is usually an adaptable person who, if his old job has been eliminated by mechanization, will readily take on a new one created by the change or by expansion. He apparently realizes that the machine will raise his standard of living in the end, and anyway he loves new gadgets and new ways of doing things. Most of the groups of technicians, experts, business directors, and the like that have crossed the oceans to see what makes America tick, would agree that my first two factors, if not the most important ones, ought to come high on the list.

The third factor contributing to prosperity, namely hard work of the people, does not receive such complete support. I talked to a German-American who was quite sure that the American worker is the laziest man on earth. On the other hand many people think he is a sort of super-Stakhanovite. I can only compare the average American with his counterpart in Britain and France, and I think the American works the hardest and the fastest. Anyone who does not agree with this ought to eat lunch at a drugstore or hamburger stand and watch the rate at which the orders are prepared and cooked. Let him ride a New York City bus and see the driver take fares, drive, give change and transfers *and* act as his own conductor by means of a large mirror. If the visitor is still not convinced, he should spend an hour or so watching a building being erected. He can do so through the convenient holes in the protective fence provided for "sidewalk superintendents." Or he could visit Madison Square Garden or a baseball game, where he will be sold hot buttered popcorn and crackerjack with a speed and intensity which are quite amazing. Perhaps the Americans are thought to be lazy by some because of their marked disinclination to use their legs for walking. Even this, though, can have a bearing on work, as I found out from my barber. "Walk," he exclaimed, "I just can't afford to do it; time is expensive. In the time I save driving to work I can do a haircut and a shave."

Lastly we come to the system, which is one of free competition. I have put this last not because I think it is of minor importance but because I cannot decide at what point to place it in the list of factors. A layman in discussing economic systems is on rather dangerous ground, but he can raise a few points. I think that as long as the excellent supplies of raw materials hold out, the free competition will work well. If there comes a time, however, when two or three important raw materials are in short supply, as in Britain now, there will have to be much more control than there is at the moment or the economy will suffer. Some emphasis should be placed on the word competition because, having seen gas and other price wars in progress many times, I know the competition is of the most vigorous type, totally different from the sort that Americans call "comfortable European competition." There is no doubt that the vigorous competition is very pleasant for the customers and it rightly cripples the inefficient. But the small business tends to suffer even if it is operated efficiently. The small business man has great difficulty in competing with the giants like Macy's and Sears, Roebuck. Usually he does so by opening his shop well before the big stores and closing it long after them. A small grocer near our apartment in New York was open from 6:30 A.M. to 10 P.M., each day except Sundays, when he was open for a shorter time. This is hard on the owner but it can hardly be said that the customer suffers. Apart, then, from the difficulty it causes the small business man, the free and vigorous competition, promoting as it has a search for more efficient methods of producing and selling and a constant effort to gain a greater turnover for lower profit per article but greater over-all profit, has contributed in no small measure to the general prosperity.

Yes, a general prosperity it is, and the American people can be justly proud of it.   A. R. B., 1951

Housing and Welfare

NEIGHBOURHOOD UNITS ᕗ In recent decades the neighbourhood community has gradually come to be considered the desirable goal to aim at—a small, self-contained community with all that it wants for its immediate needs, but forming part of a larger community which provides it with those services which alone it cannot support. Sociologists and planners, particularly in Europe, have considered that these groups should be composed of people from various social levels and from all age groups, and this has been achieved in a number of instances in European countries.

In the United States, a number of such neighbourhood units have been planned or built, particularly during the last fifteen to twenty years. Some examples are the Greenbelt towns for the Resettlement Administration—Radburn, Sunnyside—co-operative schemes like Park Forest near Chicago, private development ments like Fresh Meadows, Long Island, and the Fairless Hills scheme in New Jersey in connection with the United States Steel Company's expansion, and the Government-sponsored projects like Oak Ridge and the Tennessee Valley Authority towns. Their numbers are, however, relatively few, and here it must be made clear that I am referring, not to mere housing estates, however large, but to a complete community with shops, schools, recreation and medical facilities, churches, and preferably some form of industry planned in relation to it.

A fine opportunity occurred immediately after World War II to add to this very desirable form of development, but it was missed owing to lack of regional planning, the desire to get as many houses built in as short a space of time as possible, and the average developer's dislike of large-scale planning, which ties him down and forces him to give up, for unremunerative communal purposes, land from which he could make a good profit by high-density housing.

The examples mentioned above have not, by and large, catered to old people or to the poor, both unproductive forms of housing as far as the investor is concerned. They have been mainly occupied by what might be called the working age group drawing salaries or wages varying between relatively narrow limits in the middle range. It is, however, vitally necessary that both the poor and the aged be provided for in such projects, so that the higher-priced development can subsidize the lower and so that these two classes may take a proper part in community life and not be shut off like lepers in their own "untouchable" projects.

The lack of a comprehensive regional plan is most noticeable in almost all areas, with the result that developments have not been correlated with others in the vicinity in relation to communications, density, communal and other facilities, and appearance. It seems that this lack of large-scale planning springs from an incomplete understanding of one of the fundamental tenets of American life, one which requires much more careful thought by every citizen than it is usually given. The ideal of the personal freedom of the individual is a magnificent one, but unfortunately is not understood by a large section of the people. Freedom is not free; every man has a responsibility towards his neighbour, and failure to recognize, work for, and submit to regulations imposed for the good of the people as a whole can only result in chaos in some form or another, particularly in the complex structure of present-day life. The freedom of the individual must be subordinated to the needs and welfare of the community. To what lengths such regulations should go and where the line should be drawn is an extremely difficult question. It seems to me that they could, and should, go very much farther than they now do in the planning field in the United States.

As examples of the fields in which planning control might be strengthened or widened one might cite, firstly, the appalling ribbon development along major highways in the vicinity of towns, such as the route from Baltimore to Washington, a highly uninviting introduction to the nation's capital—rows of shacks, eating houses, bars, and garish signs, usually haphazardly placed and completely undesigned; secondly, the lack of co-operation between townships so intent on maintaining their own individuality that they will not join with their neighbours in planning for the good of the whole area; and thirdly, considering still larger areas, unreasonable variations in regulations from State to State, creating great difficulties in the development and nation-wide use of mass-produced products capable of reducing building costs.

Most Americans whom I have met have spoken with approval of some development, housing or civic, that has been well designed and laid out, and over which a strict control is maintained to ensure that there shall be no deterioration. Few, however, appear to realize that if they wish developments of that kind to be not merely isolated examples but almost universal, they can only achieve this end by a united demand and by subordinating themselves in a certain measure for the good of the community.

S. C. W., 1952

PUBLIC HOUSING ᢒᔈ With a few outstanding exceptions, public [housing] projects in the low and medium rental fields are better designed architecturally, better laid out, and better maintained than those erected by private enterprise, and therefore of aesthetically greater value to the city. Here we are faced with a basic difference between American views and those held in Great Britain, the Commonwealth generally, and the free European countries. In those countries the government or local government civil servant is a more or less permanent official, highly regarded by the general public, well paid and proud of his position. In the United States, on the other hand, many of the appointments in government service are political and liable to change with the party in power, with consequent lack of continuity and lower departmental efficiency. Moreover, in keeping with his greater individuality, the average American citizen tends to look upon a public official as a man who has not the drive to make himself a niche and fortune in this land of great opportunity, and consequently does not credit him with intelligence and efficiency or regard him with the respect that his counterparts are accorded across the Atlantic.

Is public housing necessary? Or has private enterprise provided, or could it provide, sufficient dwellings at the required rental or cost? Private development has produced some very excellent, well-built, and well-maintained projects; such, for example, as Stuyvesant Town and Peter Cooper Village in New York City, Fresh Meadows on Long Island, Parkwood Towers in Houston, Parkmerced and Stonestown in San Francisco, and others, but all of these are far out of the reach of the average slum dweller.

Granting, for the moment, that certain sections of private enterprise have been able to produce dwellings to mortgage at a weekly payment which could be paid by a fair percentage of slum dwellers, and assuming that the initial payment required were drastically cut or eliminated entirely by more liberal financing or Federal subsidy, would a complete solution to the housing problem then be provided, eliminating the need for public housing? I suggest that the answer is quite definitely "No" and for the following reasons:

Firstly, the lowest prices that have so far been achieved have been in the warmer climates where heating and insulation requirements can be cut down considerably, with consequent saving in cost. Furthermore, dwellings in this price range have mostly been built, quite naturally, on cheap land which is almost invariably some distance from the city, thereby putting an extra burden of fares on the occupant, which the low-salaried can ill afford. It seems unlikely that these prices can be duplicated in the regions liable to cold weather, or in or near the larger cities where the slum problem is, in fact, the greatest. Indeed in these latter areas a large percentage of slum dwellers must be rehoused in multi-story apartments, and there is no evidence at all to suggest that private enterprise is able to approach even the maximum allowable rental in this class of development.

Secondly, when a slum dweller is transported to a new, modern dwelling or apartment, experience has shown that a period of education or supervision, usually not more than six months, is almost always necessary in order that he and his family may learn the fundamentals of clean, sanitary, healthy life and community pride, without a knowledge of which slum conditions may again soon prevail. Furthermore, absolutely first-class maintenance of the estate is essential; otherwise this class of tenant is liable in his habits to reflect the slovenliness that he sees around him. I consider that no private developers are organized, or would be interested, to carry out a program of education of this nature on the large scale necessary for wide-spread slum clearance. This service is provided as part of their normal duties, and usually efficiently, too, by local housing authorities all over the country. It is a service for which the community at large must accept financial responsibility.

Thirdly, there is the question of whether private developers would be prepared, when it finally came to the test, to devote the larger part of their energies to producing this very low-cost type of development, foregoing larger profits on more expensive housing. It would seem, if the existing slums are to be cleared in any reasonable time, that it would be necessary for at least half the annual output of housing to be of this class, a situation very unlikely to be acceptable except during a depression.

Fourthly, low-cost housing of this kind requires extremely careful and competent design if it is not to be an eyesore, and in this field the record of private developers, with a few honourable exceptions, is very poor indeed. Public housing is producing buildings of a high and consistent standard of design and layout; all housing authorities employ competent private architects in the locality to design their schemes, whereas many private developers appear to have little appreciation of design, layout, or colour, to look upon the appointment of an expert to advise them as a waste of money, and to think that practically anyone can design a house as well as a trained professional man.

The conclusion must be that public housing is necessary—in fact vital—and particularly so at this time when slums and urban blight are growing with industry. A big effort must be made, much bigger than is being made at present, if this cancerous growth is to be not only halted but eradicated, and public housing must play the leading role.   S. C. W., 1952

PUBLIC ASSISTANCE AND "CASE WORK" ?➜ In Britain today, the necessity for a public assistance service is not questioned, and even its cost provokes little criticism; although the local officials of the National Assistance Board meet often with ignorance and misunderstanding of their job, they rarely meet hostility; they have on the whole in recent years been swimming with the tide of public opinion while their American colleagues have been struggling against it. No public assistance service can or should expect freedom from criticism, but the British service has in fact enjoyed over the last few years a remarkable degree of public acceptance and a benevolent attitude on the part of Parliament which certainly has no parallel in the United States. . . .

Superficially, the "landscape" which American public welfare presents to the eye of an enquiring Briton is a confusing one. It is often confusing to Americans themselves, even to practitioners in the field, but I think that it is confusing to the British in a particular way. Many of the laws and practices concerned have an English ancestry (beginning with the Elizabethan Poor Law of 1601), from which British public assistance seems to have made, if only recently, a wider departure than American.

At the same time many aspects of the administrative organization —administration by county and city authorities, local boards of lay persons, national participation by means of Federal grants-in-aid, subject to the fulfilment of certain minimum conditions, and so on—bear a sufficient resemblance to the arrangements which obtained in Great Britain for a long period and which were only finally brought to an end five years ago, to give one a momentary illusion of having stepped back in time rather than forward in space. But the briefest reflection and observation at once make it clear that the problem of organizing a public welfare administration in this huge country of America, this federation of forty-eight separate States, is a very different one from that which confronts the British administration, and that development could hardly be on the same lines. . . .

At this point I must say something about the "case work approach" which in America is a fundamental part of the thinking, if not invariably of the practice, in public assistance. It is a difficult subject because no two people ever seem to be quite in agreement about the definition of "the case work approach." I was often told that the success of a particular public assistance administration or of an individual social worker lay in the extent to which it, or she, had been able (in spite of the difficulties and discouragements of the public assistance job) to adopt a case work approach to it. By this is generally meant the ability of the worker to approach her client's problems as a whole, to understand, let us say, something of the impact of his economic circumstances and social environment on his personality and something of the effect of his personal attitudes on his outward circumstances, to know something of the mental as well as the physical pressures which are likely to beset people who are chronically sick, long unemployed, lonely, or rejected by their social group; in fact, the conception already referred to of a special kind of personal (or doctor-patient) relationship between the case worker and the applicant.

In a sense the entire public assistance administration in the United States has been built up round this personal relationship, and herein very largely lies its strengths and its weaknesses. It can be seen as a number of these isolated personal contacts between social worker and client fitted only quite loosely into a legal and administrative framework—this accounts both for the often admirable constructive work which is done in the public assistance field and also, I suspect, for some of the confused organization, lack of direction, and overlapping which I encountered. In Britain, on the other hand, at least since a national organization was set up, the framework of law and organization came first and nearly all the energies of the administration have been directed to streamlining the operations of what is regarded as primarily "an income maintenance service." This is a term which is used somewhat disparagingly in the United States, and even when administrative officials were prepared to admit to me frankly (as they sometimes were) that with large case loads and untrained staff they could not at present *achieve* much more than an income maintenance service, they mostly still *aimed* at the ideal of a true "case work service" and were often unwilling to admit that many of the programs they were administering are, and must be, largely concerned with the amelioration of distress rather than with rehabilitation, which I take to be the case workers' true field. . . .

If one leaves the realm of theory and policy to ask how much "service," along with money, is *in fact* provided in both countries, it is clear that the differences are not so great as the differences in attitude might lead one to expect. In the United States the most realistic administrators would say, I think, that they were trying to give all the service their staffs had time for, with the bias in favour of case work as described above; in Britain we should say much the same except that for case work we should substitute some phrase (more accurately representing our attitude and our goal) such as "trying to provide such help as a good neighbour might be expected to give." I must add here too that a very great deal of this sort of practical and good neighbourly help and advice is in fact provided, along with the cash, in the British system, whatever reluctance the officials may have to talk about "case work" or "service." Whichever the approach, the crux of the matter is to identify the case needing special attention and the kind of attention required, and having done so then the public assistance worker in both countries has generally to find some other more specialized agency to provide it. . . .

I was favourably impressed by the emphasis on rehabilitation, the real effort to "end their clients' dependency" which so many public assistance workers are making. Much thought and experiment are going into this field, and many States have made really valuable arrangements for identifying, advising, and assisting a return to work by the disabled or the "social misfit."

J. H.-W., 1953

SELF-HELP ⁊ The Chestuee is a tiny tributary of the Tennessee River which has become so blocked with fallen trees and overgrown with bushes in the course of years that any heavy storm causes both banks to be flooded and has therefore put several thousand acres of first-class bottom land completely out of use. Plans had been made to build small dams in the upper watershed, to cut the bush from the banks, and to clear the logs from the river. It was to be a co-operative job, with all the local farmers helping with tractors and labour, since almost all of them stood to benefit. But instead of the progress which I had been led to expect, little had been accomplished in two years beyond the clearing of one mile of river and a great deal of talk. My high opinion of the T.V.A. dropped several points.

A few weeks later in Georgia I saw in detail an exactly similar problem in the Settingdown Creek, a small tributary of the Chattahoochee River. Here the Soil Conservation Service had worked out in detail what profit each farmer would get if the land near the river ceased to be flooded. The farmer himself had stated what use he would make of the land—he was not told or "advised" what to do with it—and the calculations were based accordingly. When the plan for the clearing of the creek was first published, it shewed exactly who was going to get what out of it, and the relation between the cost of each part of the scheme and the expected profit from it. The scheme as a result got away to a flying start. Three small dams had already been built and seven miles of the creek cleared within a year, together with much re-afforestation and improved land management to prevent further silting up later. The local farmers were co-operating enthusiastically, which in the sphere of soil conservation was, I regret to say, certainly not the case in Tennessee. It was apparent that throughout north Georgia the idea of protecting the soil had been established for some years, while it was difficult to find any evidence of this in central Tennessee.   F. A. L., 1953

HUBERT HOOKWORM ᏽᎲ There was a health bulletin that contained all the information. It was entitled "Hookworm: A Simple Sketch for the Layman." Dr. Flesch would probably have given it the same readability marking as the Yellow Fever broadsheet put out in 1952, the backs of which many of us are still using as scrap paper. The trouble with the health bulletin was that the laymen for whom it was intended had, generally speaking, no idea that they went by any such impressive name. A panel undertook the rewriting and decided to have something that would be interesting to boys and girls. The first result was something in penny-dreadful style called "The Life and Death of Hubert Hookworm." To the literary the title said something and seemed clever. Calm consideration, however, indicated that perhaps the writers had become so interested that they had momentarily forgotten the most important rule of the writer who seeks to communicate ideas: *Remember the reader.* Testing the

new pamphlet by the readability formula showed that its reading level was still too high. So the panel got to work again and
produced a pleasant little shocker on the comic strip level. On
the title page of the leaflet was:

> HUBERT was only a little worm.
> But he looked big to Tommy.
>
> TOMMY found out how Hubert
> keeps boys and girls from
> growing strong and well.
>
> THIS STORY tells you how
>   TOMMY
>   LICKED
>   HUBERT.

Tommy was shown in the illustrations as a school lad running
off barefoot to fish for minnows, with Hubert Hookworm getting
into his foot. It went down with the school children in a big way
and they saw a boxed note at the end:

> Dr. Strong sends you this story of Hubert Hookworm.
> TAKE THIS STORY HOME TO YOUR FATHER
> AND MOTHER. They will want to read it too.

And Mom and Pop did. The fact that Hubert was written at
the fourth grade level did not stop them from reading it also.
The results were sensational. Within a month the State Laboratory cried, "Stop!" So many specimens and requests for country-
wide hookworm surveys had piled up that all requests had to
be refused for the rest of the year. That was the beginning of the
end and Hubert was well and truly licked.   F. P. C., 1953

Schools

THE KINDERGARTEN ❧ The brightest spot in American education
is the kindergarten. Here, at the age usually of five, children are

not yet involved in the grade system and the teaching is based entirely on a study of child development. Much of it is devoted to helping children to "get along" together. It is strongly in the American social tradition, delightful in its atmosphere and, to my mind, thoroughly valuable as education.

This kind of approach is spreading steadily into the lower grades, particularly the first three (which are occasionally described as primary and for which, as in San Francisco, separate schools have sometimes been built recently). I remember particularly some excellent work of this sort (a project based on breadmaking) in the second grade of a school in Compton, near Los Angeles. In this approach there are the healthy implications that the teacher is more important than the grade and that subject-matter exists mainly as an instrument to teach children to think. Indeed, I have heard Dr. Earl Kelley of Wayne University, Detroit, advance the view that the best teacher of young children will not even select his subject until, by discussion with the class, he has discovered what their current preoccupations are and has decided which can be turned to the best educational advantage.

The "project" method is often misunderstood by teachers. It is too frequently regarded as an end in itself rather than as a means which sometimes offers more scope for different talents to contribute than does following a textbook. The setting up of a project demands hard and skilful thinking to ensure that it shall be rich enough in educational possibilities and wide enough in its scope to give some opportunity for everyone to get value out of it. I recall especially as good examples the construction by junior high school boys in Macon, Georgia, of a detailed working model of a hydroelectric plant and, again at Compton, California, a project on South and Central America which required one group to report on the physical resources of the countries and another to make a rough model of the Panama Canal.   A. A. P., 1951

PUBLIC SCHOOLS AND DENOMINATIONAL SCHOOLS ⮿ An English administrator familiar with the difficulties of applying to his country the solution of the denominational school problem adopted by a country as near and as relatively like his own as Scotland would hardly expect to find in his country's practice a solution of a problem confronting a country as distant, as dissimilar, and with such different traditions of its own as the United States. And in fact the circumstances of the two countries differ very considerably. Apart from such obvious facts as the great size of the United States, which enforces a different pattern of government, and the great variety in the origins of its people, the Roman Catholics form a larger proportion of the population than they do in England, they are conscious of their strength, and they do not hesitate to use it; the Jews, at any rate in the big cities, are more numerous and influential; and there is a quite astonishing variety of Protestant sects, not to mention a profusion of more exotic cults.

Further, over the greater part of the country the public schools are more extensively patronized and are held in higher esteem by *all* sections of the community than their counterparts in England. The public schools in fact occupy a quite unique position in the affection and regard of the majority of the people of the United States and there is an influential body of opinion which thinks that all children should go to the public schools. . . . There would not be the slightest reason to suppose that the Roman Catholics, or even the other denominations concerned, would willingly give up their separate school systems. And even supposing that religious education should at some future date be given a definite place in the curriculum of the public schools, it is inconceivable, if the balance of religious forces remains much as at present, that any such measure could meet the demands of those who claim that the denominational element should permeate the whole curriculum.

At the same time the denominational school systems might

be considerably impaired if the country's economic circumstances should deteriorate. At present the churches are operating under conditions of unprecedented economic prosperity. If conditions should change, a family with limited means is going to think twice, as some obviously did in the years of the depression, before paying tuition fees and other dues for facilities which their children could obtain in the public schools without charge.

A further possible source of weakness, particularly for the Roman Catholics, is a shortage in the supply of teachers. The Roman Catholics rely to a very large extent on the various teaching orders to staff their schools. The number of those likely to be moved to seek religious vocations in the future is not a matter that lends itself readily to statistical prognostication, at any rate by a layman of a different denomination and from beyond the seas, and the opinions expressed on the subject by individual priests differ. Some, while conceding that there has been a decline in the number of postulants, claim that it is now increasing. Others say that it is falling off. Whatever the actual position now, the forces of secularism are still strong. Americans are a people who, in Mr. Alistair Cooke's phrase, "in violation of the best advice of the best English divines, . . . just don't believe that whatever is uncomfortable is good for the character"; and even for the boy (or girl) with a disposition to devote himself to the betterment of his fellows there are now plenty of alternative, thoroughly honourable, forms of social work which do not involve either the rigours or the deprivations of the religious life. Nor is it every order which has the attraction of a habit designed by Christian Dior. . . .

Whatever happens, it is to be hoped that the parochial and other independent schools will not disappear from the educational scene of the United States. The best of these schools, notably some of the preparatory schools in New England, are as good as any schools anywhere. Not a few of them, on the other hand, may leave a good deal to be desired, both in the conditions under which they work and in what they achieve. But these defects could be remedied, and, taken as a whole, the independent schools provide an element of variety which *need* not be divisive —and in this observer's view at any rate it is important that this element of variety should be preserved because, despite the heterogeneous background of the people of the United States and the very great variety in their natural physical surroundings, neither of which can be without their effect, there are at the present time so many very powerful forces at work making for uniformity in the realm of ideas.   R. N. H., 1952

FROM SCHOOL TO COLLEGE ｅｗ From grade school to the end of high school American young people, in contrast to their British cousins, have rather a pleasant existence. When they graduate they are well-developed social animals—they are in general self-confident, self-reliant, and much more self-possessed than their British counterparts, who for five years have taken an educational battering. The American at this stage is much more mature, much more at home with the opposite sex, knows the value of money (and indeed sometimes has been earning it since he or she could walk), has very definite ideas about making money in the future, and knows the rewards of success (partly from experiencing or seeing the adulation and hero-worship showered on football stars at high school). On the other hand, an American at this stage would be ill equipped to attend a British university—he is deficient in mathematics, and his knowledge of written English is poor (although he is capable of speaking and lecturing well). The American university recognizes these deficiencies and proceeds to repair them to some extent in undergraduate courses.

The undergraduate courses in American universities follow the pattern of British high school courses. There is much more "teaching" than in our universities. The student is loaded with facts and subjected to continual "quizzing." The quiz, as the name implies, is designed to determine how many of the facts given have been absorbed by the student. They are usually in the form of multiple-choice questions or the "yes-no" type. The quiz to my mind is an abomination—it encourages learning by heart, discourages thought, and gives the student no practice in writing a coherent story. It is, of course, convenient for the examiners, as it is possible to machine-grade examination papers.

R. M. M., 1950

NEGRO TEACHERS ᛒᛥ In Bibb County, Georgia, at the time of my visit, Negro teachers were receiving 80 per cent as much as white teachers. In September 1951, equality was established. There is one significant by-product of this policy, which is being increasingly adopted in the South. Within his community the Negro teacher is relatively much better paid than the white teacher in his. Since financial and social standing are closely linked in the United States, this means that the Negro teacher is a considerable figure in his neighbourhood, and this is all to the good.

A. A. P., 1951

"SPARE THE ROD . . ." ᛒᛥ I was impressed by the freedom given to children, both at home and at school, especially because of the contrast with the customs in Scotland. I caused a sensation once by mentioning that in Scottish schools pupils were punished (physically) for having too many spelling mistakes in work they had been asked to study as homework. The idea of physical punishment was horrifying enough to my American audience but the idea of being punished for not *knowing* something appeared barbarous to them. (For my part, I was equally horrified at the spelling of some of the college graduates I met in the U.S.A.) As a result of the freedom they are allowed, American children and American adults appear less self-conscious, wherever they happen to be. On the other hand, formal instruction at the high school level seemed to me well below Scottish standards.

A. B., 1949

Press and Radio

GOVERNMENT USE OF MASS MEDIA ξ❧ Mainly during the present century, three instruments have evolved for the more efficient conduct of the relations of the Federal Government with the press and—more lately—radio correspondents. They are the press conference, the release or handout, and the press liaison officer. Each has had its critics. Each has been from time to time misused. Each is generally accepted as permanent, even by those who inveigh against the use of press conferences to conceal, instead of to disclose, information; point to the wastepaper baskets filled with worthless handouts; or complain that press officers set themselves up as barriers between the press and the actual source of news.

Press relations come to much the same thing everywhere. In comparison with Britain, press conferences are more frequent in the United States, high officials easier of access, press releases more numerous, and press offices more amply staffed. At the same time, the country is much larger, the civil service is three times as big, there are 1,800 daily newspapers, none of which is national, and official Washington is served by several hundred newspaper and radio correspondents. It is sometimes said that the press conferences held by the President and other high officials are the nearest American counterpart to question-time in the House of Commons. That may be true, but the analogy cannot be carried far. The main point of similarity is that, in default of a forum to correspond with Parliament, the Administration uses the press conference and the press release for statements which here would first be made to Parliament.

As far as news is concerned the radio is on the same footing as the press: the President's press conference has been renamed "Press and Radio Conference." For the rest, one of the statutory duties of American radio is to conduct itself "in the public interest," and this has been interpreted as meaning that it must make proper provision for public information on governmental among other themes. In the thirties the radio networks were receptive to direct help from Federal agencies, and there were a considerable number of feature broadcasts which had actually been prepared in Washington. The networks now take the view that they themselves should prepare such broadcasts, and most Government departments in any case lack the staff to do the work. The effect is that there are next to no feature programs dealing directly with governmental themes or measures, as distinct from documentary and discussion programs which may, incidentally, serve the same purpose. Documentaries broadcast by the Columbia network in 1947 included, for example, "Eagle's Brood"—on juvenile delinquency, and "A Long Life and a Merry One"—on public health. The latter fitted in with the publicity of the Public Health Service. The former stimulated so much interest that the Department of Justice asked for further programs synchronized with its own campaign on juvenile delinquency. Similarly the radio networks co-operated in the food conservation program of the Luckman Committee.

The main impact of Government publicity through the radio is, however, either through talks or through advertising. Competition for network time is severe, but in practice all the four networks make time available on request for the President, and arrange that at least two of them carry a broadcast by the Secretary of State. I was told that other Cabinet members would ordinarily be carried on two networks, but below the Cabinet level heads of agencies, such as the Veterans' Administration and the Federal Security Agency, may find it difficult to get a hearing, and ordinarily the criterion would be the probable interest of the talk to listeners. Their opportunities of making network appearances are more likely to occur through participation in the forum programs which are a commendable feature of network activities. In these, the networks try to give a hearing to representatives of different important interests, including Congress, business and labour as well as the Government.

After a brief period in the thirties, when Pare Lorenz and

other gifted producers were responsible for some excellent and popular Government documentaries, the production of informational films by Federal Government agencies for domestic consumption has fallen into virtual abeyance. The few survivors of those days look wistfully towards Canada and across the Atlantic to lands where their medium seems to be better appreciated. Congress has even prevented the exhibition in the United States of films produced during the war for overseas audiences. The Department of Agriculture has the advantage of its own fully equipped Motion Picture Service, but it is limited by lack of funds to the simplest forms of production, and can rarely, for example, employ actors or orchestras. It distributes films mainly through 76 film libraries in State universities and extension services, and through its field offices, some of which have their own projector trucks. In 1946–47, 142,173 shows, with an attendance of over 12 million, were reported, but the Department thought that 25 million would be a conservative estimate of the total attendance.

There are no systematic arrangements for the exhibition of Government films in the commercial cinemas: the inadequacy of the machinery for distributing non-theatrical films is a handicap to all documentary producers. Hollywood is, however, ready to lend a hand on occasion: a documentary and some short films were produced for the Luckman food conservation campaign. There are, too, certain governmental themes which lend themselves to feature presentation. Thus the film treatment of "G-men" must have helped the skilful public relations of Mr. J. Edgar Hoover and contributed to the impression of the Federal Bureau of Investigation as an efficient machine which rarely fails to get its man. Similarly, I saw two films—one fictional, one a March of Time documentary—based on the work of the "T-men," the Treasury agents who enforce the Federal laws relating to tax evasion, narcotics, liquor traffic, etc. The Treasury had co-operated in the production of each.   J. A. R. P., 1948

GOOD NEWS ࿔ Journalists are essentially people, communicating with other people by various mechanical means. The best editors choose the best staffs and run the best newspapers. But the community which a newspaper serves also has a considerable effect on that paper. There are apparent exceptions; the English *Manchester Guardian* serves (primarily) a business community which, a priori, might have been expected to hatch a duckling rather than a swan. The international *Christian Science Monitor* is published in a city which is one of the worst served, so far as its local and conventional press goes, in the United States. But generally speaking, a newspaper's readership plays a large part in moulding it, and (though to a lesser extent) a listening or viewing audience, their pulse constantly fingered by Hooper and other public opinion experts, do obtain roughly the radio and television programs the majority desire.

Only a very great, and very exceptional editor, upheld usually by a very exceptional tradition, can force his readers not only to *take* what he thinks is good for them, but also to *like* it. And the same would no doubt hold good of the American television and radio networks if any such Titan had so far concerned himself with them.

In the last resort, what influences a newspaper reader most, of all he reads in his paper, is the day-to-day news, and the effect of this is long-term. Therefore while one can lay it down as a general law of the press that no paper which lacks a good editorial page is a good paper, it should be added that sound, balanced selection and treatment of the daily news in the news columns is the first and absolute essential of a worthwhile press. The United States is probably as well served in this respect by its minority of responsible and authoritative papers as any other country by *its* (proportionately similar) minority.   A. P. S., 1952

BAD NEWS ࿔ An emphasis in American newspapers on the affairs of the royal family, or on the quainter features of a now atypical "society" (Butler Goes Berserk, Shoots Two), at the expense of more everyday matters, seems aimed (probably subconsciously) at bolstering preconceived notions of Britain rather than presenting it as it really is. Mr. Bevan's anti-Americanism has received more space than the pro-Americanism of Messrs. Churchill, Attlee, and Eden put together. Yet this is—unfortunately—a reciprocal process. The isolationism of General MacArthur, Mr. Hoover, Senator Taft was afforded greater prominence in the British press than, as it turned out, the domestic political support for these personages actually justified. Bad news, like bad currency, drives out good.   A. P. S., 1952

AN ADVERSE VIEW ❧ During my stay I discovered only one paper with a disinterested editorial staff, and even this was biased on religious matters: I refer to the *Christian Science Monitor*. There are, of course, newspapers which are reasonably honest though partisan, for example, the *Times* and the *Herald Tribune* of New York, but the vast majority seem thoroughly irresponsible. The wireless broadcast news commentators are no better; not one of those whom I heard gave a factual report, but all of them gave a highly personal interpretation of such of the facts as interested them. Until one appreciates this situation it is rather frightening. For instance, for the first month I was in the United States I was convinced that war with Russia was imminent and that only an iron censorship imposed on the British press had prevented my learning of it sooner. After such an initial reaction, one learns to discount the commentary superimposed over the actual news and ceases to be frightened. Finally, one begins to appreciate the situation and to consider it in the light of one's views on the educational processes of the country, and there is again reason for fear. But now it is from consideration of a situation where an irresponsible and unscrupulous press is the general source of news for a great many people who, though they have acquired "learning," have not greatly developed their critical faculties and have not necessarily been trained to think. The responsibility for this situation lies largely with the editorial staffs and news commentators, for I cannot believe that they do not realize their power over opinion and their capabilities in educating people to the true facts of a situation. The argument that the general public likes tripe is no excuse for instituting a single-dish menu!   G. O. J., 1947

NEWSPAPER ADVERTISING ૨૭ No survey of the American press, however brief, could fail to take note of its advertising side. Most British visitors (particularly if they are making the meagre post-war newsprint ration at home the basis of their comparison) will patriotically declare that American newspapers carry too much advertising, and it is true that this is what has swollen them to what seems an unhandy size. Yet in a world where brotherly love has not yet dictated a communal sharing of newsprint stocks, and so long as the American reader is willing to carry a pound of newsprint about with him and chase a story through 60 or 100 pages, a holier-than-thou attitude on the visitor's part seems uncalled for. The real weakness of the business lies in the fact that the older newspaper plants were not built to print such a volume of pages, that the production process is therefore slowed (for instance, the editorials have to be written earlier) and that much of the "news" on the pages printed early has to be timeless "fudge" of no great value to the reader.

Do advertisers exert pressure on editorial policy? My liberal-minded friends will tell me they do, and I have no doubt that they are in some instances correct, particularly, perhaps, where local politics are concerned. This depends solely on the character and courage of the editor or publisher concerned. But if the vast majority of newspapers' policies tend rightward rather than leftward—as the facts indicate—and the majority of their advertisers hold similar views (and the accusation is not often that advertisers exert pressure in a leftward direction, I think) then such pressure as is exerted in the political field is probably not very important.

The whole question of why the press in the United States should now be predominantly Republican (and in Britain Conservative) is a puzzling one, not made less so by the discovery that in both countries newspapermen in the lower ranks are generally to the left of their own papers' policies. Possibly the simple explanation is that publishers are more often business men than active journalists, and that business men are more often conservative than liberal.

Nor should it be forgotten that newspapers *are* business. The left-wing experiment of publishing *PM*, a newspaper without advertisements, failed in New York partly, one imagines, because it was too extreme a reaction against the ballooning-by-advertisement process. Actually, advertisements are, in a sense, news, and there is a long tradition of the association of "ads" and editorial matter. What is important is (1) to ensure a fair ratio between one and the other, (2) not to cause readers active discomfort through inflationary bulk, and (3) to make certain (as all responsible papers seem to do) that the advertising department shall exert no undue influence on the editorial side.

I refer particularly to the example of *PM* because it seems to me that in the newspaper business, as elsewhere, sudden and extreme measures of reform, which take no account of existing social and economic mores, are likely to fail. It was suggested to me by an editorial writer on the *Sun-Times* of Chicago, another Marshall Field property, that a different policy was there being pursued, namely to build up a circulation in competition with the *Chicago Tribune* by normal competitive methods, and then, once that circulation was solid, to take a stronger editorial line of disagreement with the *Tribune*. This would be a process of years rather than months, and seems to me to have more likelihood of success than the short, sharp revolution, a phenomenon of which the public in democratic countries is wisely suspicious, whatever the motives of its instigator.   A. P. S., 1952

CHAINS AND COLUMNISTS ❧ Nobody is more conscious of his country's shortcomings, to the point of positive self-flagellation, than the liberal-minded American. And I soon learned to expect a denunciation from him of the American press as stirring as any offered by Mr. Aneurin Bevan of the "prostitute" habits of Fleet Street. Such criticism is basically healthy, because the press of both countries is certainly far from perfect. Yet it seems on the whole to be too extreme. The best newspapers in Britain and America are probably the best newspapers in the world. (I am told of formerly notable papers in South America, and I know of responsible organs in India, France, and other places. But English newspapers addressed to English-speaking readers have been for more than two centuries in a position of advantage.) Both countries have their share of dull newspapers and of bad ones, but only in about the normal proportions of human error.

Allowing for differences in geography (which, for example, prevents any one daily newspaper having a "national" circulation in the United States) and tradition (the "crime-busting" activities of the American press are nowadays, at least, much more strenuous than in Britain) I found the pattern surprisingly similar. The best papers in both countries are liberal in outlook. There are occasional respectable party organs (say, the *New York Herald Tribune* and the London *Daily Telegraph*) but on the whole, it seems to be the case that too strong a political affiliation, whether of the Left or Right, is not good for a paper. Bias is almost certain to seep off the editorial page and into the news columns.

The weakest feature of the American daily press is probably the "chain" (and it should be remembered, where British comparisons are being made, not only that we have "chains" of our own but that the mass-circulation national dailies in Britain are, in effect, the same thing). It is bad, in my opinion, because an integral feature of the system is the distribution, from some central bureau, of "canned" editorial material. In the Hearst group, this centralized direction is strict though perhaps less so than it was under the present publisher's father.

In others, such as the Scripps-Howard chain, local editors are given more discretion (though the question of which Presidential candidate the group was to support was a "headquarters" decision). But whether the rein is tight or slack, the fact remains that the reflection of local opinion on the editorial pages of "chain" newspapers is restricted, and that this is regrettable. The British Government can and does take careful cognizance of the editorial views of independent provincial newspapers, as reflecting feeling in the area they serve. The Federal Administration is denied this assistance wherever and to the extent that a "chain" is operating strictly. It is a strange paradox that many an editorial complaining of over-centralization of government in Washington must have been distributed through the country from a Washington editorial bureau.

All this is not to say that the *whole* system is bad. When it simply cuts administrative costs and permits the publication of a newspaper where there would otherwise be one less available, it seems beneficial. But to cut costs below the line required for editorial independence is likely to remove the backbone from a newspaper. And there is no justification at all for the "chain" proprietor who is not content with making a profitable business enterprise out of it, but must also needs impress his own political views on a wide variety of communities with whom he stands in no personal relationship.

From this subject it is a natural step to the question of the syndicated column. Here again there is a bright and a dark side. Ideally, syndication, like any other method of artificially standardizing opinion, seems undesirable. But in so large a country as the United States, with one central government, it is better that the smaller and poorer newspapers should share a Washington correspondent than that they should have none at all—indeed the same principle applies, on a lesser scale, to State capital correspondents, who are often shared among several papers also.

There are a number of responsible and able columnists operating from Washington and New York.

There are also the irresponsibles, among whom X ("the only newspaperman with the courage to tell the truth," as an admirer described him to me) and Y are pre-eminent as writers and thinkers in Billingsgate—ersatz Menckens with none of that professional insult-monger's finer qualities. It is here alone, that the responsibility of the American press as a whole falls seriously short of the necessary standards. Editors and publishers whose papers regularly carry columns of semi-slanderous inaccuracies are pandering to depraved tastes just as truly as vendors of pornography; and to reply to criticism with "Ah, but the public wants it" is no better answer in one case than the other. It is noteworthy, I might add, that the two Eastern columnists mentioned above have not penetrated, in any force, at least, to the West Coast. . . .

The "attractiveness" of the editorial page is a subject I have heard discussed by many editorial writers on both sides of the Atlantic. It is known that a readership of 28 per cent or so is all that can be expected for editorial matter compared with 72 per cent for the comic strip "Blondie." But in one particular the American editorial page is handicapped by comparison with the British. Partly because of the larger size of the American papers, and partly perhaps as a result of some older tradition based on greater difficulties of communication in a bigger country, the editorial page has a low priority (priority being used here in the newspaper case-room sense that it is "put to bed" early) and is printed earlier than in Britain.

As a result editorial writers often do not write so "close to the news" and their editorials do not possess that immediacy which is or should be one of the attractions of a British editorial page. It has been argued that the American system allows more time for research and a considered approach, but the finished products do not, on the whole, support this theory.

A. P. S., 1952

NEWSCASTS ৯৯ The radio was a more common source of news than the newspapers. The breakfast-time bulletins were always heard and were the major means of information. The newspaper, when it arrived later in the day, was dismissed with little more than a cursory glance, and it was, in any case, twelve hours or more behind the radio. To understand why people in the Middle West are sometimes so confused about foreign affairs, one must listen to the newscasts of small radio stations.   H. A. H., 1953

HOMESICK ৯৯ I just longed for the BBC.   J. R. G. B., 1949

Language and Popular Culture

A GOOD MEMORY ৯৯ A redheaded gentleman who said his name was McLennan tapped me on the shoulder and said that his forebears came to America about 1600 and had never spoken to an Englishman since. I said it was wonderful we could still understand each other after three hundred and fifty years.

C. H. W. M., 1948

PITFALLS OF LANGUAGE ৯৯ One of the first striking features of the spoken language is the remarkable uniformity of usage and of accent over wide areas and, even more striking, the comparative absence of class differentiation. The difference between a well-educated Chicagoan and a less well-educated one lies chiefly in the restricted vocabulary of the latter, rather than in any lack of grammatical accuracy on his part. Neither does the uneducated man seek to overcome his poorer powers of expression by the use of language socially unacceptable to his "betters." Not that swearing is unknown, but it seemed to this observer that the snatches which floated to him across the streets of Chicago were if anything more acceptable than the corresponding flotsam that might be gathered in, say, London. There are, of course, one or two pitfalls for the unwary in this matter of "bad" language. One or two words fit for quite refined English ears become the cause of raised eyebrows in the States, while more than one English blush has been called up by one or two items of the American vocabulary considered fit for polite and even mixed company. There is no need to illustrate the point. It does not often lead to serious embarrassment, partly because some Americans are aware of the facts, and partly because the American curiosity overcomes all barriers when such a *faux pas* is committed, so that the matter promptly becomes the subject of free and friendly discussion.   D. V. O., 1951

Is THE LANGUAGE DEVALUATED? ᘐ Another feature of American speech and writing is the undue (to English ears) use of superlatives, a habit connected, I think, with a most important aspect of American life. It is the capability for enthusiasm and warmth, virtues which are either possessed to a singular degree by the American people or are lacking to a similar degree in the English. The curious feature of the situation is that many Americans like to be thought of as hard-headed; while many Englishmen look down from a great (and totally imaginary) height upon the unseemly ebullience of their cousins. It is this enthusiasm, though, coupled with a genius for work, which is the great creative force in the States, and which often achieves far more than the more balanced and analytical viewpoint which is at best sterile and at worst disillusioned. Perhaps it is a virtue which can only survive while it is possessed more or less unconsciously, without being explicitly recognized and labelled; if so, long may American business men continue to describe themselves as hard-headed.

But if this enthusiasm is virtuous, its effects on the language are far from beneficial. The smallest size toothpaste tube available in the States is Medium-Sized. Beyond this we have the Large Size (still of quite modest proportions) followed by the Giant Size and then, for a large tube, by the Jumbo Size. Finally, if something really large is required, the vocabulary, which has been strained too far, breaks down and one is constrained to ask for the Economy Size. This amounts to a re-definition of the words "large," etc., which would be moderately legitimate if they were required only in this kind of context. But a financial report, for example, which attempted to use the newly defined words by speaking not of "a large deficit" but of "an economy deficit" would justly be accused of an attempt at confusion. Yet the word "large" is losing its force, and it has no universally applicable substitute.

A certain disrespect for words is implicit in the attitude just described, and this disrespect is manifested in other, and more objectionable ways, one of the chief of which is illegitimate back-formation. "What did you think," asked one of my American friends, a very bright philosophy student, "when the pound was devaluated?" There are quite a number of instances of this kind of treatment, of which I may quote "to eventuate" (to happen) and "to slenderize" (to slim). And, in the same class of verbiage of unnecessary length, "in the event that" (if), "is located" (is), "prior to" (before), and "end result" (result). How do such curious formations pass into such common use? The only theory which I can advance is that language is treated as a servant and not as a master of expression.

Certainly the more remarkable of the above concoctions appeal to the ear as being outrageous long before they appeal to the intellect as being unnecessary or uneconomical. The Englishman attaching a certain divinity to words is well content to say only those things which the words say easily and of themselves. The American may have a vision of new concepts to which the language must be made subject.   D. V. O., 1951

SELF-CRITICISM ᎒᎙ Two main trends are noticeable in American life; first, the development of culture (in the humanistic sense of the word); and second, the progressive debauching and degrading of public taste. That two such trends are inconsistent does not mean that they may not co-exist in the same society. By the development of culture is meant the appearance of mature artists and art forms, and of places in which they may meet, work, and be exhibited. For the first half-century of independence, the United States was a cultural province of Europe. Even in the second half of the 19th century, although great American writers (Hawthorne, Melville, Mark Twain, Whitman) were beginning to appear; although Emerson had hoisted the flag of literary emancipation from Europe; although Whitman invited the Muse to "migrate from Greece and Ionia," and "cross out please those immensely overpaid accounts"; in spite of all, America had not shaken itself loose and still could not think of itself as other than a cultural apanage of the Old World. A few artists were able to express themselves genuinely in native terms; the rest yearned towards Europe. The writer and artist came in search of "atmosphere," the wealthy in search of paintings, statuary, antiques, titled husbands.

The growth to maturity was a slow one, but the United States is now a mature—not to say static—nation. Its libraries, art collections, universities, orchestras can take rank with the best in the world. Its painters, poets, novelists, playwrights, musicians, have no need to feel apologetic to Europe. Indeed, where such figures—Henry James, Whistler, T. S. Eliot—once were drawn to Europe, it is now the Europeans—Auden, Isherwood, Aldous Huxley, Thomas Mann—who are drawn to America. The semi-exiles like Hemingway and Henry Miller are home again. Gertrude Stein of Paris, France, is dead. It seems a long way back to the remark of the American lady, Mrs. Touchett, in Henry James' *Portrait of a Lady*, that "they all regard Europe over there [America] as a land of emigration, of rescue, a refuge for their superfluous population." It is true that the United States, especially the Northeast, still defers somewhat to Europe, in particular to England. The visiting lecturer is a great draw, and there are always some books by British authors to be found on the best-seller lists. But on the whole American culture stands upon its own feet, interested in Europe as a partner, not a guardian or parent.

The parallel tendency towards vulgarization has been so much written about that it hardly needs further comments. The interest in sadism and violence, evident in Disney cartoons as well as in the novel and the cinema; the evergrowing emphasis upon sex and romantic love; the increasing importance attached to the corpse in funeral rites; the capture of radio by advertising, and of the cinema by similar forces; the lowness of educational standards, and the contempt for the "expert" (except in business) and the "highbrow"; the combination of narrow Puritanism with a soaring divorce-rate; all these and other matters are familiar reading to Europeans. One item will do to summarize the process. Babe Ruth, a great baseballer and national hero, died recently after a painful illness. Within two hours of his death, printed copies of a valedictory song that had been prepared for the event were mailed all over New York City to such people as are concerned to appraise or plug popular music. To such revolting ends does a worship of commercialism in society lead. If songs about a dead hero sell best while the headlines are still announcing his demise, then obviously the song should be written before the death, and kept in readiness.

But if we are to take this incident for text, it should also be noted that many people were shocked by it; and that one "disk-jockey," commenting upon the recording of the Babe Ruth song, asked his listeners not to buy it. In other words, the fight against vulgarization is waged in the United States as fiercely as anywhere. It was Mencken, an American, who wrote so scathingly of the "Great American Boob." No foreigner has attacked the country more violently than the American, Philip Wylie. No society is so interested in itself, or subjects itself to so much examination. The task of the intellectual or the social critic is harder than in Europe, but it is not shirked.

Europeans do, I think, yield too easily to their "Athenian Complex." Is Europe so much freer from materialism, from vulgarization? It was an American who said to me that, in one sphere, lend-lease consisted of the supply by America of vulgarity to England, in exchange for culture. He was unfair to his own country. Europe is following the same path as the United States, with every sign of enthusiasm. Indeed, in some aspects she is in the lead. The pushing and unlettered millionaire, so often taken as an American type, is a British invention; who was more flamboyantly "American, self-made," than Robert Hudson, the Railway King? And what example of gregariousness can the United States, the home of folksiness, put up to match Butlin's Holiday Camps in Britain? What American newspaper can compare, in circulation or content, with the *News of the World?* Western civilization as a whole is faced with a dangerous cheapening of standards. It seems unfair to blame America, when we are all involved. The common European error is to equate American popular tastes with European intellectual ones. (Nor, of course, am I saying that popular tastes are necessarily bad. Some popular tastes in America—as that for square-dancing or New Orleans jazz—have great vitality.) The intellectual is perhaps more hemmed in, here in the United States, more apt to be stigmatized as "radical" (or un-American); yet his work stands up to scrutiny. Let the European match "lowbrow" likings on the two continents, and then note, as he must, that Europe craves the American popular idiom, whether expressed in music or movies or literature of the *No Orchids for Miss Blandish* genre. The same process, I imagine, is at work in South America; the "Yanqui" is resented for his prosperity and his "materialism," but the American ethos is being accepted. The era of the Common Man is on the way everywhere, and the uncommon one must survive as best he can. M. F. C., 1949

POPULAR SCIENCE ⮞ Much American advertising and semi-popular writing of the *Reader's Digest* type seemed to me to reflect the faith of the American people in science and in exact and numerical statements (or what they believe to be such). For instance, in Baltimore I saw on sale "pH Gin"; this is sold in what look like chemical flasks, and its labels show a scale (coloured red for acid and blue for alkaline) of pH values of different drinks, indicating that this gin, unlike various other drinks, is neither acid nor alkaline in reaction. I doubt if this approach to the public would be considered profitable in any country but the U.S.A. However, hypocrisy is one road to virtuous behaviour and I believe that the advertisers who have popularized exact statements rather than generalizations are now gradually being compelled to confine themselves to true exact statements; and this is in part through public opinion which they themselves have helped to generate. Certainly the Federal regulation in the field of food and drug advertising is much in advance of what we have in Britain.

But while its exploitation is the most conspicuous sign of the public's faith, I consider that to be only a symptom of the state of the popular mind; that is, its faith in measurement and its conviction that science can provide the answers to material questions. Some grasp of scientific method (or at least of its logical component) and a modicum of factual scientific knowledge are necessary components of the culture appropriate to this age, and I think that in America the popular conviction shows that at least one essential step in the right direction has been taken.   B. A. D. S., 1952

CULTURE: A MISSIONARY SERMON ᘒ My own notions about America before setting foot on her soil form a closed chapter in my past neither relevant nor pleasing to recall. The widespread notions entertained today by a good number of Britons, while no more pleasing to observe, are highly relevant. American hospitality, generosity, and technical ingenuity seem to be universally accepted as indisputable facts, and a returning Fellow has no difficulty in persuading people that he found these virtues everywhere and in everyone, abundant and flourishing. But culture, taste, and judgment? No, despite the Boston Symphony Orchestra, the *New Yorker,* and the text of the Constitution, the Briton sadly shakes his head. Culture is the almighty dollar, chromium-plating, fake Gothic, and taking cine-shots in Athens. Taste? Why, everyone knows that Americans put ice-cubes in their beer, and would spurn Taylor '29 if there was Coke around. Judgment? Look at the witch-hunting and the Hiss trial.

But the task is not hopeless. "All right," you begin, "so there are 52 million motor vehicles for 150 million people. That doesn't mean that possessing a car is the be-all and end-all of the American's existence; he's about as proud of it as you are of that canteen of cutlery—it's a comforting and pleasant necessity. And his ice-box and his wife's washing-machine aren't things he boasts about either, because they too are just basic necessities, part of what people expect from life along with policemen and street-lighting and not things they hanker after so that they can feel they're little J. Pierpont Morgans. Many Americans are as genuinely shocked and astonished to hear that you haven't got them as *you* are to hear of the pavement-dwellers of Calcutta.

"Americans drink Coke (and that I'll grant you is something of a mystery), but only where you drink lime juice or lemonade or ginger pop; there is proportionately far more good table-wine drunk in America than in England. And by the way, the only ice-cubes I've seen in beer were in a distinguished London hotel —served to two puzzled and dismayed Bostonians.

"As for appreciation of the arts, well, I'm afraid I can't tell you much about what most manual workers think; how the Pittsburgh factory worker gets his fun is a closed book to me, but I imagine his favourite retreat is very little less elevating than the crowded pubs and street-corners of Birmingham and Sheffield. And a couple of things do stand out in my mind. I've looked at the queues outside the Metropolitan Opera House, and they were no more made up of Columbia dons than the Albert

Hall queues are of London ones. I remember, too, the sixteen-year-old son of a New Haven rooming-house keeper who owned and played a collection of serious music on records that would have been the envy of an Englishman of taste three times his age. I remember, also, a minor teachers' training college in Muncie, Indiana. Muncie is a little country town, in its proportions and in its economics rather like Louth in Lincolnshire. With a half-hour to spare, I wandered into this training college and to my surprise found it had an art collection housed in several excellent galleries. There were some Holbeins, a Giovanni Bellini, and a couple of Andrea del Sartos—the only ones I've ever happened to see; and as it was vacation time, the dozens of people wandering through must have been just townsfolk.

"If I tell you about the opera, music, and drama in Ann Arbor, a midwestern city of only 40,000, and of its packed public lectures on political policy, religion, philosophy, and international problems, you'll say, 'Well, of course; you'd expect those things in a big university centre.' But there aren't just three or four big university centres in the United States, you know; there are ten big ones and a score of smaller ones *in the Midwest alone.* Oh yes, and before you raise that old one about the commercial radio and soap operas, did you know that many of the universities themselves have high-powered radio transmitters broadcasting programs unsurpassed anywhere in the world? Besides, up and down the country, there are several big independent radio stations (like New York's WQXR) which put over material with a quality familiar on the Third and with a warmth familiar on the Home.

"I nearly forgot the witch-hunt. I'll grant you that it has existed and in fact still does exist, just as I'll grant you some other poor features of America, like the dreary postal and city transport services; but don't forget that there have been a few witches worth hunting. And if you with your political maturity have got the idea that McCarthyism is a nation-wide philosophy, how can you blame some American readers of the *New Statesman* if they run away with the notion that England is rabid with Bevanism?"   R. Q., 1952

Sports

FOOTBALL IN THE SOUTH ⪬ Each New Year's Day two of the most successful southern football teams meet in New Orleans. The game is a great social event; everybody goes to it, if only to wave at friends, or merely to sit in the open air and cool one's head after the parties of the previous night.

This year Texas and Alabama were the contestants. When we got to the stadium, half an hour before the game began, it was already almost full. It was a gay, noisy, cheerful scene. The sun was shining, the crowd laughing and talking. All over the field padded and helmeted gladiators were practising, going through motions with a ritualistic seriousness, some kneeling and sprinting, others bobbing and side-stepping, others again flinging themselves down in adroit tumbles—thirty or forty players to each side. And each side had its band—the Texans in orange cowboy costumes and black Stetsons, the Alabamans in a gaudy comic-opera uniform. Each band had its drum majorettes, high-stepping in brief skirts, their movements as ritualistic as the players', or as those of the cheerleaders—bareheaded youths in sweaters who postured, leaped, and clapped. In the crowd it was easy to pick out the Texans by their wide-brimmed hats; everybody seemed to be wearing a favour of some sort. Overhead in a benign blue sky, three or four airplanes towed streamers advertising a restaurant or a brand of drink. This was Dixie, but not the nostalgic kind, mummified charm; it was the New South, still proud to be Dixie, prouder still to be the Lone Star State (in the case of the Texans), but cheerful, energetic, prosperous. A fur-coated crowd of whites who had dined well. What of the Negroes? My ticket had specified that it would admit only a "member of the Caucasian race." I supposed I was a Caucasian, and on entering found myself among Caucasians. Over on the far side of the bowl, in a separate section, sat some of the non-Caucasians; the Negroes.

There was much of the South and of the United States in that scene. Regionalism: a strong sense that this was Dixie at one of its own festivals. Negroes—the dark slice in the cake of the spectators. Optimism—the crowd happy and each side loudly confident of victory. Energy—how loudly they all sang and cheered! Prosperity—one had only to look around at the new clothes, or the big new cars outside the Bowl. Showmanship—how highly organized were the bands and cheering sections. Sentiment—how reverently we all rose and doffed our hats to sing "The Eyes of Texas Are Upon You," and the Alabama songs. Gadgets—people with pocket radios, listening to commentators on other games while watching this one. Specialization—players trained for certain tasks, and brought on and off the field continually to fulfill them and then make way for the experts needed next. And above all, colour, spectacle, good humour—the atmosphere was irresistible, and Denis Brogan is right in likening it to that of the Greek Games, as a ceremony in which the whole community comes together, to sing, to cheer, to admire the feats of fit young men in a moral equivalent of war.   M. F. C., 1949

SOCCER ও The rules of American soccer vary little from those used in England, but substitution should never, in my opinion, have been allowed to creep into the game. The would-be player should possess a working knowledge of Spanish in his academic equipment, since that is apparently the language common amongst players and referees—for all I know, it may be Portuguese, because a Brazilian in the team never seemed to be at a loss for words. That I have no such linguistic talent did not matter because it is more common for players to talk *at* a goalkeeper than *to* him. It interested me to hear that the popularity of soccer on the West Coast is increasing. One reason for this lies in the fact that the game lends itself better to television than does football; the bold, mobile geometric patterns executed by the "soccos" are fascinating on a screen (and the cameraman cannot be fooled by a wily quarterback). If America would field representative soccer teams (or conversely and less likely, Britain would adopt football), Anglo-American relations would perhaps improve further. Our two countries have all too little in common in the way of popular sport.   R. E. D. B., 1951

CRICKET AT CORNELL ⁊ As a result of the American War of Independence, cricket has never flourished in the United States, although the climate is more suitable than it is in England. I gathered that the Americans have developed a similar game which makes less use of guile and is a little faster than cricket, and which requires some of the players to wear over their heads a sort of wire cage or muzzle, designed, I suppose, to protect the wearer from stones and bottles or to prevent him from biting his opponents. Cricket clubs are few and far between, and Cornell's nearest rivals were Rochester, whom we thrashed in our first encounter on their home ground.

The return game at Cornell was the subject of great preparation and publicity. By some fluke there was no baseball game arranged for the Saturday of Alumni Weekend, and so the cricket match was scheduled as alumni entertainment. We waived our right to charge gate money for the sum of one hundred dollars which we got from the Alumni Secretary and which made us solvent. A large crowd of alumni and wives gathered all over the field of play and had to be swept off before the game could begin. We had arranged with the local radio announcer to give a commentary on the match over a loudspeaker, but although he was an intelligent and upright American, his knowledge of the game was meagre and there was some confusion and a little inaccuracy now and then. However, all went well before a docile, uncomprehending crowd who were pleased to be informed at the end that Cornell had maintained its unbeaten record.   H. D., 1952

V. Envoi

THE ANGLO-AMERICAN ᙄᎤ Is it meaningless to speak of being an Anglo-American? The answer to this began to take shape when I met someone, a few weeks after my return, who had never heard of William Faulkner or Scott Fitzgerald. Later, it was a man who knew of Washington, D.C., but had never heard of the State; others thought the letters T.V.A. had something to do with television. My reactions would have done justice to an American born and bred—or almost so! I was beginning to learn what it means to be an Anglo-American. I recalled those other occasions when I had told my American friends of James Bridie, explained that the University of Glasgow had not been founded by a Victorian tea-planter, and the B.B.C. was not "in the pocket" of whichever political party happened to be in office. The experience had now come full circle.

The home-coming of the Anglo-American is characterized by his secret dismay that others have not been privileged to range so far and that it is often difficult for them to see more than their half of the picture. It is with something of this in mind that I speak of the dilemma of return. On the one hand there is the amazing ignorance and the alarming gaps in our knowledge of America and the American people and on the other the fascinating story of America to tell—or rather epic, as I have chosen to call it. There are the differences between us more difficult to cross than the Atlantic, and yet similarities which speak of a

218

past in common and point to the hope of a future in common. There are the criticisms of American capitalism and resentment of her position of world leadership which must be answered with a sense of admiration for a country which in recent decades has assimilated two revolutions; in the social sense, that of the welfare state and in the international, that of abandoning isolationism.

In all this, if one is honest with oneself, there is the tendency to slip back into accepted ways of thinking while the urgent need is to foster that sense of partnership and the need for communication which have just been awakened. These are the horns of the dilemma which face the Anglo-American. If he owes his existence as such to the experience of a Commonwealth Fund Fellowship, he is well fitted to grapple with them. More than that, he will welcome the opportunity—for it will be his personal response to the many kindnesses of the Fund and a relevant though distant salute to a much-loved country and people. D. G., 1951

TEXT ࿐ No one can understand another country only in happiness. W. A. B., 1952

SUMMING-UP ࿐ If, as a young would-be theologian, I may be allowed to indulge in one final reckless generalization, I would say this: if it is true that in Britain we are too sure of ourselves and too self-satisfied, it seems to me no less true that America, for all its resources and all its resourcefulness, is a country which is basically not very sure of itself and not so self-satisfied; and that, to a theologian, is of course the greatest praise. R. A. S. B., 1953

Index of Contributors